The Powers of Addiction

Finding Freedom in Acceptance and Recovery

By Cesar Wurm

Foreword

By Tom Counts

What makes this book so special is to see the depths that someone can go to in order to hide their addiction. Cesar presents this in an open, brutally honest format that bears his weakest moments. It takes true courage to admit some of these actions and I do not know many people who have that kind of strength, but it shows through in brilliant honesty.

I have known Cesar since January 2002. When I started as a Senior Sales Manager at The Sheraton Atlanta Hotel. Cesar was fresh out of the Management Training Program, and kudos to Brad Rahinsky for having the wisdom to promote him to the Sales Department as an Account Manager. After my first week on the job, Brad asked me to "Look out for Cesar" as he "needed some mentoring but will surely be a superstar". Cesar came to me with questions, and as an industry veteran, I shared my views on crucial hotel sales topics, including the importance of room block guarantees, attrition, and cancellation fees. This was at the time when the Revenue Directors reported to the Director of Sales and Marketing, so we got to discuss why rates were where they were one week, and much less the next week. Discussing the importance of Holidays, City Wide Demand, and building relationships with Corporate Clients, which can make or break a hotel.

As with any time that I played the role of teacher, I really learned more than I taught because it gave me an opportunity to get other people's opinions as well, and then sometimes I would share with Cesar, an update, based on popular opinion from the powers that be. As I read the book, flashbacks of certain events came back to me, and it all clicked. Cesar was working me, just as he had worked everyone else along the way, and I was not aware. It is rare that anyone has pulled the wool over my eyes to such an extent, but for sure, I was fooled. Once, in all of that time, we had an event at the hotel, and when the event was over, we took some of our premier clients to the Hotel Bar for a few post event cocktails. The next morning, during our daily "Standup Meeting" we all went through the business that we had planned for the day, our General Manager called us all out by going over the bar tab from the night before. At the conclusion of a good flogging, he said "Who drank 14 Jack and Cokes", we all kept our mouths shut, and I suggested that the bar staff might have put some drinks on there from people that were not really with us. But, I knew that Cesar was drinking Jack and Coke, and I did not count his drinks, but I did tell him later that I was rather impressed with 14 drinks after a night of partying. We had a good laugh.

At the time that we started working together, Cesar was single, very single, and I was married, and I would say, happily married. We would go out as a team for celebrations from time to time, and I would always get an update on Monday morning as to the shenanigans that the younger single guys in the office were up to. The raw success that they were having in Atlanta, where single straight men were at a premium, was truly amazing, and Cesar and his co-worker Mark were great story tellers, and I have to say, it was entertaining to say the least. I am looking forward to reading that book: if it ever gets published.

As Cesar grew in his career, we had ample time to discuss strategy on how to build up a market, and he was really gifted when it came to building his business base and creating loyalty beyond reason. He was my counterpart, and then got a director's position at another hotel and then after a couple of years, came back to be my boss. What was great is that we thought about business in a very similar way and had just about zero conflict when I reported to him. It really was one of my favorite working relationships ever. We were both trying to put the best business possible into the hotel, and we were getting to be very good at it. All while, behind the scenes, Cesar was going through the battle of his life.

At some point in the middle of everything, I was suddenly a single parent, and I moved to Boston and worked remotely. As remote working was not much of a concept back then, I wanted to stay at the hotel 2 weeks a month, so that I could stay ahead of things, and Cesar and I became roommates in a great 2-bedroom 2 bath apartment in Buckhead. Now that we were both single, all I can really say is that till Cesar met Laura, craziness ensued. All good stuff, but never did I have any clue that he was struggling. After a year or so of that, we got the T1 speed and technology to a point that I only came down to Atlanta for site visits, but every time I was in town, I got the chance to catch up with Cesar, and never did I have any clue that his situation was going from bad to worse. At some point in that time, I gave up drinking as I had 100% custody of my two daughters, and had to be sharp, and at the time, I told Cesar that "no one has ever screwed up their life by quitting drinking" and we had a really good laugh.

Over the next couple of decades, we kept in touch at least once a month or so, and we spoke about so many things, and I never had a clue that he was struggling. Cesar was great at what he did, and he was great at hiding his addiction. He was getting promoted on a regular basis and deemed a total success by everyone in the hospitality industry. There was a point that we were speaking about 10 years ago when he shared with me that he was thinking about quitting drinking, and I shared that "no one ever screws up their life by quitting drinking" and we had another really good laugh. Shortly thereafter he quit drinking and became a mentor to so many people who are struggling with addiction. He also chose to be a leader in the struggle and share his experience to help others. Displaying a bravery that I do not have, Cesar has made an impact in our industry, and has been a role model to many who needed a role model who is human, and relatable.

I urge you to invest some time in reading this book, to see what is possible with a positive mindset. It is an amazing story, and through it all, I had no clue till I read it in print.

Preface

Addiction. A fatal disease that is vastly misunderstood by those suffering from it and those impacted by it. Addiction will continue to destroy lives for generations to come unless we increase our awareness and openly talk about it.

It does not discriminate. Rich, poor, black, white, gay, or straight, addiction will present everyone with the same opportunities and will always be there for you as the most loyal companion you could ever have. As a society we mismanage and ignore the number one cause of accidental death. It is time to stop managing addiction through the criminal system. Addiction is a health issue and should be treated as such.

I am writing this book because it is my calling. On my path to recovery, I began to realize that one of my purposes in life is to be a driving force and a resource for others to better understand addiction through my lenses. As an addict, I have an opportunity to share with the world my experience and show how someone presumably "normal" and raised in a family and environment that is privileged when compared to most of the world population could become one. Furthermore, by helping other people I am helping myself—every addict does. My goal is to shine some light on this topic and have a positive impact in the journey of changing the perception and misunderstanding of addicts. There is a preconceived notion about addicts, their backgrounds, and how they got to where they are.

In my opinion, there are many great resources for addiction and substance abuse, but most of these are focused on the recovery process. I strongly believe this is a very necessary service for addicts. However, we need to create more emphasis on prevention. We should do a much better job getting a message out to parents, teenagers and young adults about this disease and the many factors involved that can contribute to someone becoming an addict. We need to overcome the taboo that addicts are bad people or that they choose to become addicts, among many other false and/or uneducated assumptions.

The process must start with addicts like me. We need to be brave and come out of "the addict closet." We must share our experiences with people in hopes for them to learn from us and to prevent people from becoming addicts themselves. I understand the fear that many addicts may have to make their struggles and experience public. As I began writing this book, I was still in the addict closet. Although my journey to addiction and how I lived are not something to be proud of, I *am* proud of the resilient person I have become today. My sobriety journey has given me the strength and skills to overcome any obstacle that comes my way. I am tired of saying "they" should do something about it—now is the time for *me* to do something about it.

If we as addicts don't open up and share what we have experienced so people can better understand addiction, who will? No matter how much the medical community continues to better understand and spread the message, people will not truly accept or digest the information unless it is substantiated through real life experiences.

The best way I can compare it to would be for your parents to tell you not to do something because it is bad for you. We all have been there and likely thought something along the lines of *Well, they don't know what they are talking about. I know better. This would never happen to me.* Or my favorite, *I am different.* This is likely the thought processes the vast majority of people will have if information is not shared by addicts themselves. While one will never be able to overcome all skepticism, it helps to demonstrate that someone with a good family, stable finances, great education, and professional success like me can be an addict. You don't have to live under the bridge to be one—however, many addicts will eventually end up under a bridge, in prison, or at the grave. It is just a matter of time.

I am not an expert in addiction, nor a medical professional. This book is not intended to create a new theory on what addiction is, how it works physiologically, or how to diagnose or treat the condition. I am certain some of my statements are not supported by any group of experts or medical findings, and I am ok with that. I don't want to offend anyone, but I most certainly will, and honestly, I don't care. This book is a channel to share what I know better than anyone else in the world. My journey, my learnings, and my understanding on living with this disease.

I hope this book can contribute something to you or to someone you love. No one has to go through this alone. Together we can save lives by becoming aware of our judgment of this disease and those who suffer from it into understanding.

I began this book in 2015, at 36 years of age, newly sober, with a beautiful wife and daughter. It has been interesting to reflect on my journey and ask myself where and how it all began. There is no clear answer. I wish it would be easy to pinpoint a time in my life where there was a turning point and there, I was a changed person, drinking uncontrollably from that day forward.

While I don't have all the answers as to why and how I became an addict, there is some good information provided by the medical field and sobriety literature (AA, etc.) that helps me understand some of the reasons. The bottom line is that addiction is a complex disease. To some addicts it is enough to understand that it is a disease and just move on; but personally, I wanted to know a bit more than just accept that it is the case without any reasoning or explanation whatsoever. This is a big part of my life, so it was very important to understand how I got here and how I can successfully remain sober. So, I began with a simple question. What is the definition of addiction?

In simple terms, addiction is a chronic disease of brain reward, motivation, memory, and related circuitry. I know I am oversimplifying it, but the brain basically categorizes alcohol as an essential part of our survival therefore overriding any attempt of "warning signs" or impulse to control it. Your brain sees it as a necessity just as defending yourself when you feel as if you are in a do-or-die situation. The best definition I personally found so far is from AA. It explains that an alcoholic is someone that continues to drink despite it having a negative effect on their lives.

I found that while my addiction is a chronic disease of the brain supported by my genes, it was fueled by my emotional underdevelopment. I internalized everything, I held everything inside, did not share my feelings and when I did share it was always "filtered." I am an expert in rationalizing my emotions vs. letting it be. It was like adding fuel to the fire. Interestingly enough, I found through many of my interactions with addicts that emotion usually plays a big role as a contributing factor to the disease.

There are several risk factors that contribute to someone's propensity to develop addiction. The more risk factors someone is exposed to, the greater the chances that he/she will become an addict. Some of the factors are genetics, repeated substance use, disruption of healthy habits or support system, and the inability to deal with feelings in a healthy manner, among others. Knowing what

I know now, there are 3 key areas that I believe to be the contributing factors for my journey to addiction. **They are my biology, environment, and development**.

Environment is not about global warming or air quality, but about the outside influences an addict can experience such as stress, family and friends, quality of life, and peer pressure, among others.

Our environment—social, cultural, and psychological—can increase the risk of developing addictive behaviors.

Social factors, such as peer pressure, can influence an individual's decision to use drugs or engage in other addictive behaviors. For example, if a person's social circle consists of individuals who regularly use drugs, they may feel pressure to participate in drug use to fit in or be accepted. Looking back, I never felt as if I was coerced or pressured into consuming alcohol, but I also did not avoid being around it.

Cultural factors, such as attitudes toward drug use, can also influence an individual's risk of addiction. For example, if a culture glorifies drug use or portrays it as a normal part of life, individuals within that culture may be more likely to experiment with drugs and become addicted. As a teenager this was the case in my circles with drinking as you will soon find out. One of the biggest misconceptions is when parents assume that if their teenage or young adult kids drink around them (i.e., they are better off drinking at home under my supervision), this will lead to controlled and responsible drinking. In fact, several studies suggest that these teenagers and young adults are more likely to become alcohol abusers. One clear indicator of this is how it impacts Europeans more than most cultures.

Psychological factors, such as stress or trauma, can also contribute to addiction. For example, an individual who has experienced significant trauma—this could be several small traumas or a big trauma—may turn to drugs or other addictive behaviors to cope with their emotional pain.

Part 1 of this book examines my addiction through these 3 lenses (my biology, environment, and development). Part 2 presents the 4 Pillars of Sobriety, while Part 3 concludes my story by delivering the Powers of Addiction that come from choices and experiencing enlightenment. To highlight the most powerful moments of my journey, my stories go back and forth in time instead of following a chronological order. I hope each and every reader can learn from my stories, as it is never too late to break the patterns of addiction.

Table of Contents

i. Chapter 1: My Daily Routine

ii. Chapter 2: My "Lucky" Day

iii. Chapter 3: A Party of One

iv. Chapter 4: The Wake-Up Call

v. Chapter 5: Awakening

    a. 5.1: Psychological Approaches

    b. 5.2: Lifestyle Changes

    c. 5.3: Building a Support Network

vi. Chapter 6: Acceptance

vii. Chapter 7: Gratitude

viii. Chapter 8: Community

ix. Chapter 9: Healthy Habits

x. Chapter 10: Family Influences

xi. Chapter 11: Choices

xii. Chapter 12: Inner Nirvana

Part 1: The Three Factors for My Addiction

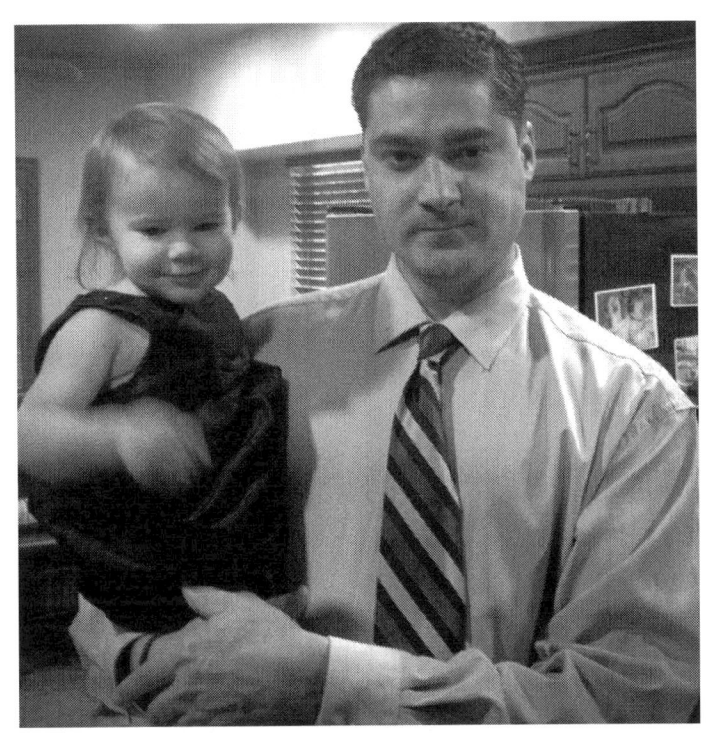

Me and Gabby in San Antonio, 2012 when my drinking began to intensify. Besides having gained weight, my face was puffy, and eyes were constantly glassy – a trait of being under the influence.

Chapter 1: My Daily Routine

I drank all day and night, nonstop.

It was 2012 and I was working as a Director of Sales & Marketing in a hotel, living in San Antonio, Texas. On my way to work I would stop by Whole Foods and buy a bottle or two of organic red wine. I always bought a specific brand of organic wine not because I cared about being "green" but because it was cheap. I could easily justify a $2.95 charge on the credit card bill as breakfast at Whole Foods if my wife, Laura, ever questioned the frequency and amount of charges.

Every plan I had and every action I took was about alcohol and how I could keep getting it.

By 7am I would have had at least half a bottle of red wine, and sometimes even a whole bottle. I drank some on my way to work, and then had a good amount in the parking garage before heading into the office. Every time I bought the wine at Whole Foods, I would get an empty coffee cup from the store so I could fill it with wine and take it with me to the office as I started the day. Who would ever guess that instead of coffee I was sipping red wine? I knew that even if people thought the color seemed strange or possibly caught a whiff of the scent, no one would ever think that Cesar would be having wine early in the morning since who in their right mind would do that? This was my routine, and by doing it every day, I had no change in pattern or behavior to make anyone suspicious.

Once my bottle or bottles of wine were gone – usually before or right after lunch – I had to be creative to get more alcohol. Since Laura took care of our finances, I could not go to a bar or liquor store to get more alcohol. I could not go to Whole Foods again. How could I possibly justify two daily trips to the grocery store, especially when the hotel offered us lunch at a low cost?

I was obsessed in my quest to get more alcohol. *Why don't I just hit the hotel minibars?*

As Director of Sales and Marketing I had access to sales showroom keys and always had a reason to go to the guest rooms. We had to show guest rooms to a client, double check the cleanliness prior to a showing, verify a particular room view, or take a quick picture to send to a client. Once I was in the room, I would hurry to the minibar looking for the small bottle of vodka. I went after vodka because it was the one with the least amount of smell, and because I could refill the empty bottles with tap water, seal the bottle well (both the cap seal and the label over the cap that guarantees the bottle was not tempered with). By the time a guest or the minibar attendant realized that the bottles had been tampered with, there would have been many key entries after mine from housekeepers to guests, so the odds of someone ever finding out or tracing it back to me was very slim. I was willing to take this risk even if it meant being caught.

After the Whole Foods wine and the minibar vodka I would usually figure out a way to get one of my co-workers to go with me to the hotel bar around 4:30pm to have a drink before heading home. My MO was to order drinks with the most amount of alcohol without calling attention to it (my favorite was a dirty martini straight up) so the buzz would not suddenly dissipate by the time I got home, and by then I would be able to have some beers and wine to keep the cycle going. It was not unusual for me to do some hidden garage drinking in between the drinks inside our home. I never wanted Laura to realize I was overdrinking, so I drank what I deemed to be acceptable in front of her and then figured out how to get more alcohol without her seeing it.

While crazy, this used to be my daily routine.

Biology: My Inheritance from My Dad

According to the National Institute on Alcohol and Alcoholism, genes are responsible for about half the risk of alcohol use disorder.

Research has shown that genetic factors account for approximately 50% of an individual's vulnerability to addiction, with the other 50% being attributed to environmental factors. The specific genes that contribute to addiction risk are not yet fully understood, but there is evidence to suggest that genes related to the reward system, stress response, and impulse control are involved. I will share a little more about it later in this book from my Biomarker Evaluation Report.

I was born with genes that were a contributing factor to my alcoholism.

Since I can remember my dad has struggled with alcohol and without a doubt, I carry the same genes. I recall moments of my dad's experience with alcohol when I was a child like it was yesterday. The memories are very vivid and painful. Today, looking back, it is interesting that once I accepted I am an addict, the biggest resentment and anger I had was toward my dad and his drinking.

The fear and insecurity I felt as a boy and as an adolescent are still very much alive. I am not 100% sure, but I am fairly certain my drinking was much heavier and more out of control than my dad's and I was causing the same if not greater pain to my wife as he did to my mom prior to her passing. I was on the same road to inflict as much if not more emotional pain on my daughter (she was a baby/early toddler, so she possibly already experienced unconscious fear and insecurity as I was always drunk around her). This is how deceptive this disease can be. I was mad at my dad for something that I was doing to a greater extent. It is crazy; I was in major denial! My state of mind was so blurry and delusional that I made justifications for my behavior.

The greatest dream of an addict is to consume alcohol or the drug of choice recreationally, as a "normal" person can. I tried many ways to control my drinking such as drinking only on weekends, drinking no hard liquor, having a glass of water in between drinks, and limiting myself to no more than two drinks a day, among others; however, it always failed. While I could manage to stick to my rules for a while, eventually the disease would creep up and conquer me every single time. I learned through a lot of trial and error that addiction is an illness that cannot be overcome just with good intentions or desire. To win against this disease there are a lot of areas in life that need to align and stay aligned. It starts with the acknowledgement that there is a problem, the understanding that you can't drink like most people, and changes in your actions, behavior, circle of influence and environment.

Environment: My Beginnings in Brazil

I grew up in Araraquara, Brazil, a small city of 250,000 people located a couple of hours from São Paulo. I was surrounded by a great group of friends who lived in my neighborhood. We were very tight from an early age and would play in the streets after school and on the weekends. I'd leave the house after breakfast and come back for dinner, spending the days kicking soccer balls, creating dirt bike tracks, and playing hide and seek—a lot of outside time and a lot of camaraderie among 10 to 15 boys just a few years apart from each other.

My childhood was a good one; not perfect but good in comparison to most. My parents did their best to raise me and my older brother, Alexandre. My mom was always very loving, positive, and giving while my dad was the disciplinarian of the family. When you think of a traditional hardline German, that was him. Tough, rigid, and fairly uptight. Of course, he loved us and did his very best to raise us and give us a good education, but it was a methodical approach.

Because of my dad's struggles with alcohol, my environment throughout my childhood and adolescence wasn't always the best and wasn't always stable. Some days were great, and some were complete misery mixed with fear.

Development: My First Sip of Alcohol

This is how one of the main risk factors began at an early age for me. The earlier it happens in life; the greater one's vulnerability becomes.

I don't exactly recall my first sip of alcohol; but I know without a doubt it happened way too early. When I was probably 8 years of age, I was with all my cousins having a sleepover at one of their homes when, in the middle of the night, I sneaked into my uncle's alcohol cabinet to sip his orange liqueur. It tasted so good—like one of the best desserts I have ever had. It was also not unusual for me to sip from my dad's beer mug (one of the traditional German beer mugs). At the time, he drank warm beer and while the taste was bitter and nothing like the orange liqueur it did not stop me from going back to it time after time.

Powerful Lessons

- Obsession is a sign of addiction. If you're planning days around drinking, gambling, drugs, or any other addictive activity, you have a problem.
- Good intentions and desire fail to overcome addiction. Winning begins with the acknowledgment that there is a problem.
- The earlier in life you are exposed to an addictive behavior, the more likely it is you will become addicted.

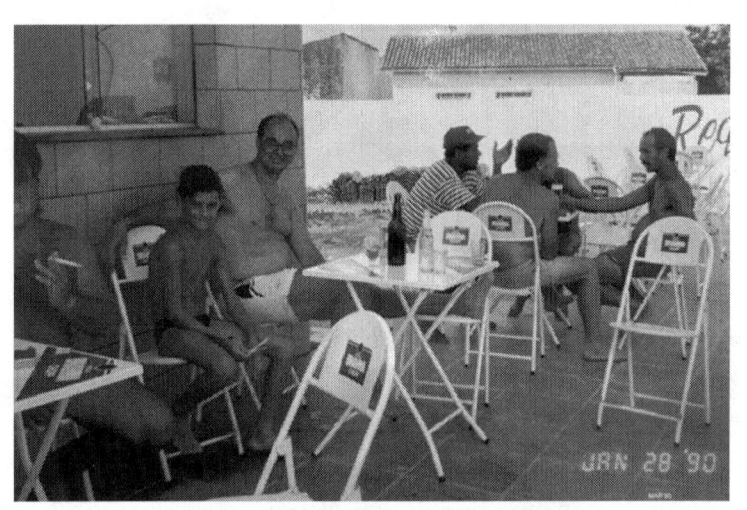

Me and my dad somewhere in Brazil on vacation.

Chapter 2: My "Lucky" Day

In the early summer of 2005, I was flying down the road, listening to Guns N' Roses and driving erratically when I made a left turn on a red light. Out of nowhere, a cop car appeared right behind me with his sirens and lights on. I continued to drive like a maniac, refusing to pull over. Eventually, I stopped, as I knew that sooner or later, he would catch me. I was only a couple of blocks from home which Laura and I just purchased. Even though I was very intoxicated I knew deep down this was not good and things would change from here on out.

This policeman who pulled me over happened to be the gentlest cop I'd ever met in my life. I don't recall much of the interaction and conversation, but I do recall my hands being cuffed and then being brought to the back of the police car. It was a horrible feeling. Besides feeling the cold hard metal pressing against my wrist—this part still feels very vivid to this day—it felt like my life was over. So many things were going through my mind. One of them was that I would most likely lose my job.

Once I was in the back of the police car, the cop asked me why I was trying to run away and what I had been doing beforehand. While I don't exactly recall all our conversation, I know that we got to know each other a bit and then he asked me where I lived. I told him that we were just a couple of blocks away from my house and that my fiancé was waiting for me. He began telling me that getting a DUI would have a huge impact on my life, not only financially. Consequences would include the DUI staying on my record for several years and following me everywhere. Then he turned around and told me something to the effect of: "You are a good kid, and I really don't want you to get a DUI. This is your lucky day. Is there a number I can reach your fiancé so she can pick-you up?"

Wow, what a relief.

Biology: Biomarkers

This is in part an extension of the brief mention I made earlier in the book about the Biomarker Evaluation Report. It enhanced my knowledge as it relates to part of the biological factor in addiction, though I am far from being an expert. My intent with this section is to take what can be an intimidating and complex topic and break it down into layman's terms, making it a little more approachable. As part of this quest, I've researched more about the biology of alcoholism and specifically the genes associated with addiction in the hopes to highlight how they can be so influential in someone's addiction journey.

One example is the DRD2 gene, which codes for a dopamine receptor in the brain. Variations in this gene have been linked to an increased risk of developing addiction, as well as a decreased ability to experience pleasure, which may lead individuals to seek out addictive substances or behaviors.

In simpler terms, the DRD2 gene is like a blueprint for creating a specific type of lock (a dopamine receptor) in the brain. This lock is designed to fit a key called dopamine, a chemical that plays a crucial role in how we experience pleasure and rewards.

Now, imagine if this lock (the dopamine receptor) is different in some people because of variations in the DRD2 gene. These variations can affect how well the lock works. For instance, people with certain variations might find it harder to feel pleasure from everyday activities because their locks don't work as well with the dopamine key. This reduced ability to feel pleasure can lead them to seek out stronger, more intense experiences, like using addictive substances or engaging in addictive behaviors, to try and get that feeling of pleasure.

Variations in the DRD2 gene can make some people more prone to addiction because their brain's reward system doesn't respond to pleasure as effectively, leading them to seek more intense sources of pleasure.

Building on this understanding of the DRD2 gene and its impact on pleasure and addiction, it's important to consider the effects of chronic drug use on the brain. Research has shown that regularly using drugs can lead to significant changes in the brain's reward system, the very system we just discussed, which is influenced by dopamine and its receptors. These alterations can also impact the brain's mechanisms for controlling impulses. What this means is that individuals who use drugs for a prolonged period may find it increasingly difficult to stop, even if they have a strong desire to do so. **This difficulty is not just a matter of willpower; it's a direct result of the changes in their brain's wiring and chemistry.** Furthermore, these changes can interact with genetic factors, like variations in the DRD2 gene, creating a complex interplay between genetics and environmental influences in the development and persistence of addiction.

Since I became sober in December 2014, understanding these genetic factors has been a desire for me. I've done sporadic research during the years, but only recently have dived into the latest science. In early 2023, I was listening to the Wired for Addiction podcast with Dr. Higgins, who discussed the recent progress in the science of addiction and how genes and biomarkers influence our behavior, and the common genetic markers of addiction. Discovering one's predisposition can be empowering, particularly when it comes to optimizing mental health and overall wellness. Armed with this knowledge, individuals are better equipped to achieve sobriety and ultimately lead healthier, happier lives.

After hearing Dr. Higgins speak, I was thrilled. Her insights opened a door for me to gain a deeper understanding of my personal journey and edged me closer to the answers I had been seeking. Immediately after the podcast concluded, I reached out to Dr. Higgins's team. Following several enlightening discussions, I chose to proceed with her Biomarker Evaluation Report and her tailored recommendations. Alongside the insights from my DNA test, Dr. Higgins guided me through six months of life optimization coaching where I had the opportunity to gain further understanding on my addiction and even having gained unexpected learnings such as that I should stop eating gluten because of some of my genetic make-up that is prone to inflammation.

Environment: The Death of My Mother

Up until recently, I believed that "trauma" had to be one big tragic event. While this is definitely one way to experience trauma, exposure to "little t" trauma can cause just as much if not more emotional harm than exposure to one big traumatic event. Ultimately, anything that causes distress, fear, and a sense of helplessness can qualify as trauma. And, when I was 12, I got a "big t" trauma.

When I was 12 years old my mom passed away from a cardiac catheterization. It was a standard, relatively low risk procedure, but my mom seemed to have had a sixth sense that something would go wrong. There were a few signs such as when she told our neighbors that she would never move into our new house, even though construction was only four months away from completion. Another instance happened a couple of nights before her procedure, when I noticed my mom cleaning and organizing my and my brother's closets, and I asked her what she was doing. She replied that she wanted everything organized "just in case."

The day that we drove to São Paulo ahead of her procedure is a memory that is still very vivid in my mind. My mom, my brother, and I sat in the back seat. A driver from the company where my dad used to work drove us, so my dad sat in the front passenger seat. The drive is about four hours. My mom and I were always very affectionate towards each other—I loved to feel her touch, receive her hugs and kisses (this form of affection is ingrained in me to this day, and I am conscious of that as I can annoy my daughter and wife from time to time with my quite touchy feely way of demonstrating affection). As we were together at the back seat, I was able to spend time in her arms and lay my head on her leg for what it seems like a good amount of time. I can still fill as if it is today when I was touching her legs and could feel the mix of her soft skin and the recently grown hair from a couple of days without shaving. I don't recall much more of the drive until we got dropped off at our cousins' house. My brother and I would stay there while my dad would go with her to the hospital.

I will never forget the last time I saw her. At our cousins' house, we got our bags out of the car and said what was supposed to be a temporary goodbye. As the car was driving away, she turned around and gave the biggest and warmest smile that I have ever seen while waving goodbye. This is a very powerful memory that still replays in my head as if it were a movie in slow motion—unfortunately not one with a happy ending.

I don't exactly recall how long the procedure and her stay at the hospital was supposed to take. The next evening, our extended family was all together at my aunt's house when my dad called to check-in. He spoke to my uncle and said that he would come and visit us for a bit while my mom still there so my uncle went to get him. When they got back, my dad walked into the living room, took my hand and my brother's hand, sat us down and told us, "Your mom passed." Boom—it was like I had gone insane. It felt as if I was having the worst and craziest nightmare, something completely surreal, while being numb all at the same time. It broke me down.

Without a doubt, her unexpected passing marked the most heart-wrenching period of my life, a profound trauma that, in the absence of adequate emotional coping strategies, significantly fueled my struggle with addiction.

Experiencing the loss of a mother at a young age is a profoundly traumatic event for a child, one that can leave an indelible mark on development and overall well-being. This loss often leads to deep-seated emotions like grief, sadness, and an extreme sense of loneliness. It can also, in certain cases, impede the child's capacity to form healthy attachments in their future relationships.

Studies have highlighted that children who face the loss of a parent during their formative years might be more susceptible to a spectrum of adverse effects. These include:

- Mental health problems such as increased risk for depression, anxiety, and other mental health issues.
- Behavioral problems such as aggression, defiance, and hyperactivity.
- Poor academic performance as they may have difficulty concentrating, completing tasks, and staying motivated.
- Substance abuse as a way of coping with their emotions. They may feel a sense of numbness or escape from their pain by using drugs or engaging in risky behaviors.
- Relationship difficulties as they may have difficulty trusting others and forming healthy attachments.

It's well known that experiencing the loss of a parent at a young age can have a huge impact on a child's growth and overall well-being. Children who go through this type of loss need all the support and resources they can get, to help them handle their grief and adjust to their new reality. Unfortunately, not dealing with this kind of loss the right way can lead to some unhealthy behaviors later down the line. And as you can imagine, that was my case.

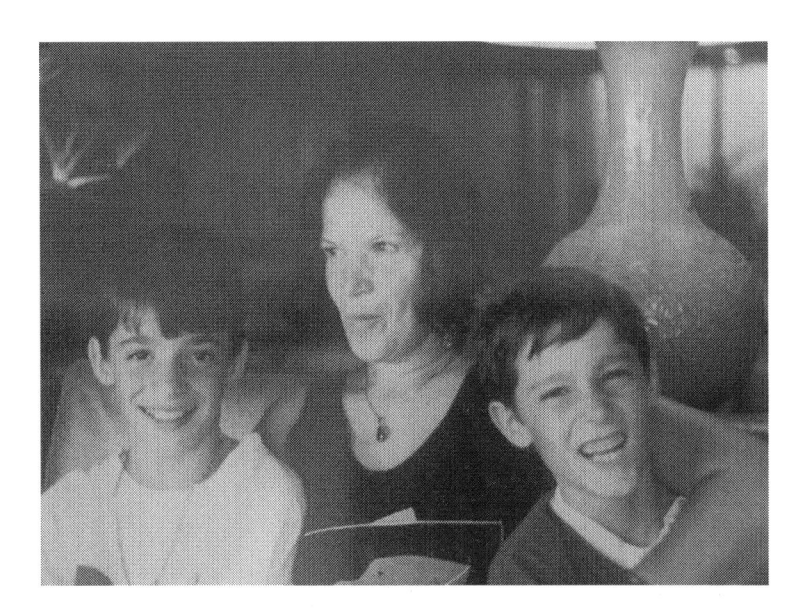

My bother Alexandre, our mom and me. Picture from the late 80's or 90 at the latest.

Development: My Early Drinking Career

I think it is fair to assume that most people accept the fact that drinking while you are not fully developed is not a good idea, hence the legal drinking age. Growing up in Brazil, while there was an official drinking age of eighteen, it was fairly normal and socially accepted for someone to drink underage. Very few places or parties (if any) enforced it in the early 90s; now it may be a different story.

As you know by now, my drinking career started very early. I recall having sporadic alcohol pre-adolescence consumption like taking a sip out of my dad's beer mug, but when I was about 13- or 14-years old drinking became a habit. Silly me at the time thought of it as a "healthy" habit and a sign that I was a man. I was tough—I could handle alcohol. Drinking became almost a daily occurrence at this early age from going to little bars ("botecos") to play pool, drink after school and going to all the clubs and parties I could.

Not too long after my mom's passing, my dad hired a tutor to keep my brother and I focused on school. He wanted to ensure we had the support we needed to complete homework and get good grades. It was an intense and long tutoring plan from 2pm to 6pm every weekday. I just hated it. I no longer could play with friends after school and my lack of appreciation for school just went ballistic overnight.

However, there was a much bigger change in the household when my dad decided to remarry less than a year after my mom's passing. Now that I am grown, I can understand his thought process, especially knowing how he is wired. He was always hyper focused on doing everything he could to provide and support my brother and me with whatever he perceived as needed so that we could have a secure future.

During his business trips, my dad used to go to several countries as the company he worked for sold orange juice across the globe. Throughout the years he got the opportunity to travel quite a few times to Asia and developed a great deal of respect and admiration for their culture, specifically for South Korea. Not too many months after my mom passed, my dad connected with a South Korean friend of his in Brazil and asked if he could help him find a wife. Someone who would be loving toward his two boys, be able to provide us with a good support system and also provide companionship to him.

My dad's friend came through on the ask and introduced him to Chong Hee, who became our stepmom. While she was wonderful, she was presented as an immediate solution to our situation, which made it difficult for my brother and me to accept, and we rebelled. I know that my dad had the best of intentions but perhaps not the best approach on bringing his vision to life. As hard as it is, I don't want to judge, blame, or criticize him for it as I know his heart was in the right place and he was just as lost as we were.

The day we met Chong Hee, we traveled to São Paulo, which was about four hours from our home. As you would expect, it was an awkward situation for my brother and me, but I venture to say that most likely it was most difficult for Chong Hee. When my dad introduced her to me, he said, "Cesar, this is your new mom." Boom—another bomb had just dropped, and it killed me inside. She quickly realized the poorly delivered message by my dad and immediately spoke out, "No, I'm not replacing her, don't say that." Throughout the years I learned that speaking out firmly as she did was not in her nature and having her say that was a temporary relief to the pain it caused, and also showed me her heart and her good intentions as she was understanding of what my brother and I must have been going through.

Soon after we met Chong Hee, the four of us went on trips to Campos de Jordão, São Paulo, and other places around Brazil, allowing us to get to know her better before she moved in with us. She was always very sweet, caring, and respectful.

While the trips were helpful and allowed us to get to know her, when Chong Hee moved in there was a lot of friction and I became very resistant to the situation. Not because of her or who she is but because I felt as if she was "replacing" my mom, the person I loved the most.

Teenage years can be challenging under normal circumstances, and this situation just exacerbated my rebellion, anger, and disbelief in how the world could be so painful and cruel. The next couple of years remained very bumpy at home mostly because of my rebellion and pushback. I pulled away and relied on unhealthy habits to bring normalcy to my life and what I thought was inner peace.

Eventually, as time passed, I let my guard down and embraced Chong Hee in my life. She has always been nothing but an amazing person and looking back I feel bad for the pain I caused her. I was always angry and resistant to her care and love, creating a barrier between us. She came into a completely new family, under very tough circumstances and, with a very different culture. I am sure it was just as hard for her, if not more. After a couple of decades, I finally had the courage to apologize to her for all the pain I caused her. Of course, she was very understanding.

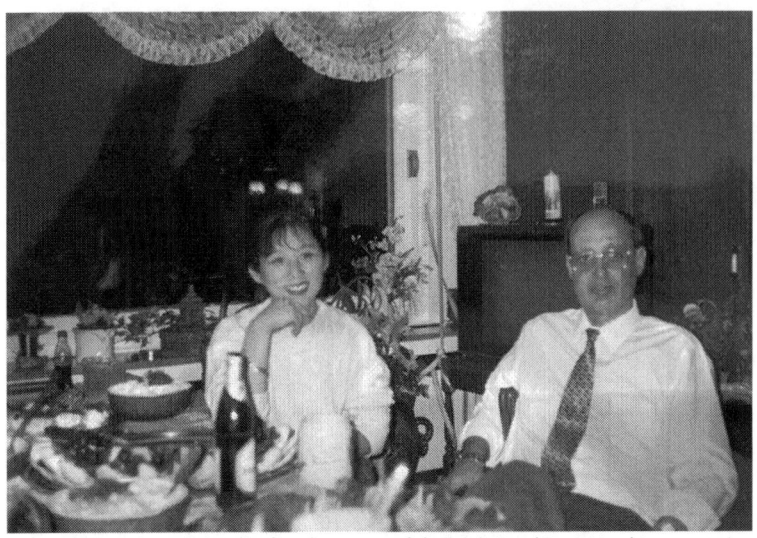

Chong Hee and my dad at the first few years of their relationship visiting his parents in Dortmund, Germany.

Consequences Versus Habits

When I was pulled over in 2005, I was fairly intoxicated, so when the officer asked for Laura's cell number so she can pick me up and avoid DUI, instead of giving her number I proceeded to give my cell number and the phone was in my car. He called a couple of times and told me that unfortunately there was no answer, so he had no choice other than take me downtown and book me. My world collapsed; I had been so close to avoiding a DUI.

As he was about to drive toward the station, I suddenly saw Laura's white Passat appear. She parked across the street and walked toward the police car. She was very worried about me as she knew I was drunk, she said, and as it was taking way too long for me to get home, she had decided to look for me. She could not reach me on my cell, and she began worrying that I got into a car crash. As she continued to approach the cop car screaming at me, the cop stepped out of the car to calm her down and told her I just had too much to drink. He reassured Laura that everything was okay and that I'd be able to go home with her. I was let out with a ticket for running a red light.

I got extremely lucky.

I woke up the next morning on the sunroom couch, so I knew that all the flashbacks of the sirens and police car were not a dream but an actual event. Laura and I had a serious talk. Clearly, she was very worried about me and what could have happened—after all, we had just bought the house and we were planning to get married the next year.

For any non-addict, this would have been the wakeup call necessary to change habits and reduce drinking greatly and of course never get behind the wheel under the influence.

But not for me. In my mind, this was an isolated incident.

Addiction progresses very quietly. Little by little it begins to overpower you. Usually when someone begins to suspect that something might be wrong, chances are that you are already in serious trouble. It is a very confusing period because you're so focused on alcohol, you lose sight of everything else in life. Even subconsciously, you may know that you have crossed the invisible addiction line, but you are so isolated and there is so much shame and fear of the slight chance you may be an addict, not to mention the terror of eventually confronting it.

During this time of my life, I wanted the consequences I was experiencing to change without changing my habits. It is the definition of insanity. Doing the same thing over and over while expecting different results. This is when my double life really began. I portrayed myself as someone and something I was not and projected what I believed people wanted and expected from and of me. I was digging myself deeper and deeper into addiction while trying to do the best acting job of my life—at times it was an Oscar worthy performance. While there was this huge turmoil and pain inside, I worked very hard to project happiness, contentment, and peace. I was on the autobahn of self-destruction.

After my "get out of jail free card," I continued with my usual drinking habit. My career continued to flourish. Laura and I married in 2006, just as we had planned. There were many more red flags along the way, including our wedding. I was drinking beers before the wedding with my friends reminiscing the "good old days" and of course there was no holding back at the reception, where I got hammered on caipirinhas—the traditional Brazilian drink that we were featuring for our guests. The last picture of our wedding is of us leaving on the white classic Rolls Royce to our hotel, and you can see in my eyes how wasted I was.

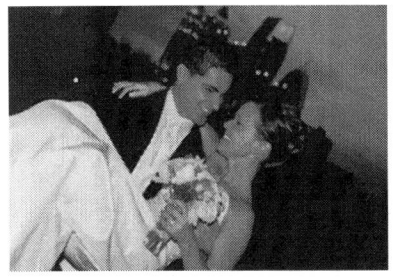

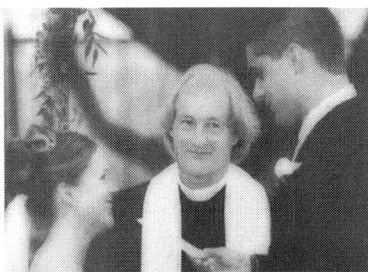

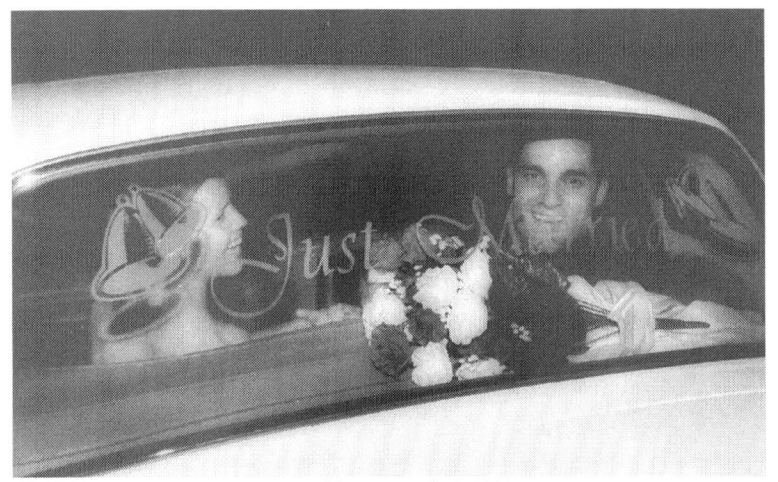

Our wedding on April 1st, 2006

Despite my heavy drinking our relationship was great. Life was beautiful. When Laura and I began dating and during the first years of our marriage, we were not planning on having kids. We wanted to enjoy our youth, have fun, go out to dinner every night if we wanted to and travel freely and spontaneously. However, in our fifth year as a married couple, we decided to have a baby. After all, what else would we have to look forward to as we grew old together? The life we were living was good and fun for the time being, but we wanted our lives to have meaning beyond just the two of us.

We were blessed with a beautiful little girl we named Gabriella. What a joy! For some reason I always wanted a daughter, and we had this adorable and healthy baby in February 2011. Being part of her birth was the best emotion I had ever experienced in my life. When I held her and smelled the purity of her breath, I felt an overwhelming warmth and joy and could not hold back the river of tears coming through my eyes. I grew up as a Catholic and as I became a teenager I pushed away from religion and never had gone back. I was spiritual, but not religious, and when I held Gabby immediately after she was born, I got all the assurances I needed that there is a higher power and miracles are possible. She was a miracle.

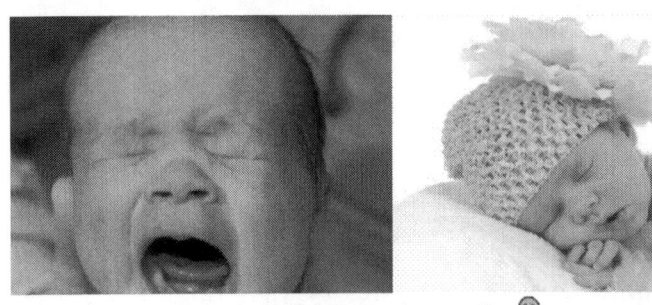

I don't think she was happy at first 😊

As we got settled in our hospital room—we would stay there a few days until Laura healed from the cesarean—I went out to grab a bite and get a couple of well-deserved beer mugs. Laura was with her mother, and I left my wife struggling with pain and the stressful and emotional roller coaster of being a new mom and trying to breastfeed. Instead of being aware of it and being present for her, I was concerned with how I could bring alcohol into the hospital room, so I wouldn't have to forgo my drinks or create excuses to leave the room often. I know it must be very hard, if not impossible, for a non-addict to understand this kind of thought process.

When a drink should have been the last thing on my mind, it was the first. Looking back at this moment, I feel so ashamed, sad, and guilty of my actions. I'll never forget an Oprah show where George W. Bush briefly discussed his alcoholism and said: "I realized I was falling in love with alcohol. Alcohol was crowding out my affections for my wife and my daughters." So true—that was me. You begin to plan all your actions, activities, and reasoning with the end goal of consuming alcohol. I was constantly thinking, *How can I do or accomplish something while being able to keep on drinking?*

My drinking intensified substantially immediately after Gabby's birth. I don't have a tangible or scientific explanation but perhaps it was the memories of my mom or the change in our couple dynamic. Everything was new and different, and with change usually comes stress. Perhaps that was my refuge and way to escape my emotions instead of learning my new surroundings and focusing on this important and wonderful journey that was beginning in our lives.

Another very important factor that fueled my addiction to alcohol was my inability to be in the moment. Throughout my life I always set goals for myself and once I achieved them, I had to set new ones. It was a never-ending quest.

Having goals and striving to do more can lead to amazing outcomes, but I was trying to find happiness and a sense of worth from external sources and not from within. No matter how much I achieved or over-achieved, I still felt an emptiness inside.

My constant chase of the next way to prove myself led me to the next big change in our lives. As Laura and I were struggling to find our footing as new parents and get a "new normal" established just three months in, I was offered a new job. And not just a new job. It was a relocation halfway across the country, from Atlanta to San Antonio, Texas, pulling my wife away from her family and the ones close to her. It sounded like a great idea at the time because it was a distraction from my alcoholism and pain but today, it hurts just thinking about it. Part of my reasoning at the time was that I now had a family to support (Laura had been a teacher and now would be a stay-at-home mom), so I justified the move with the fact that I really had to focus on my career growth. In reality, all I was looking for was to fill the emptiness in my chest and run away as cowardly as I could from my slow but steady downward spiral, hoping it would be like pushing a reset button.

The move to Texas could have been one of the best or the worst things ever that have happened to us. While it was super painful and a crazy time in our lives, it helped us get to where we are today, and I really believe everything happens for a reason.

So, with a new job locked in we moved from Atlanta to San Antonio in May 2011.

Things went okay at first. We were living at the hotel, and I felt excited about the relocation until a few weeks into the job. I quickly realized that I made a mistake. Not because it was a bad opportunity, but because I was just as miserable, if not more, as I'd been in Atlanta. Little did I know that the emptiness I had was not caused by geography, job, etc. but because of how I was living inside the world of an alcoholic. I was lonely in a completely new environment. But it was too late; I'd signed a two-year contract and if I broke it, I would need to repay our relocation expenses, which was not an option. As I was stuck in this situation, I hoped that if I kept plugging away, things would improve little by little as time passed. We eventually bought a house and began to settle in our new town where Laura could build a new group of friends. But I was still alone in my misery.

The unhappiness and stress I began to feel from my decision to move us to San Antonio was very heavy. I began to withdraw from Laura. I did not want her to know or feel that I made a mistake moving us to Texas (even though she knew it), so what better remedy to numb all those feelings and emotions than with plenty of alcohol?

At this time, I could have been classified as an alcohol abuser, but this experience and what was to follow solidified my destiny as an alcoholic if I had not already been one.

Even though Laura was swept up in taking care of Gabby and trying to get some stability in her new environment, I could tell she was beginning to realize that something was not right. I was distant, cold, almost soulless. When I look back at my pictures during that time, I can see the glaze in my eyes—a clear display of being under the influence.

Whenever Laura would question me if I had been drinking, I would firmly and convincingly lie, stating that I had nothing to drink or sometimes saying that I'd just had a drink before heading home with a friend. I'm ashamed of the lies and I'm ashamed of turning the situation to make Laura feel guilty or question herself so she would back off and not find out the truth. I would play the victim and say that she suffocated me and at times I just needed a way to escape from her pressure, that I could never have a drink without being given a hard time. So basically, in my mind, it was her fault that I lied when I lied and not because I had a drinking problem.

This went on for months. Up to this time, as I mentioned, I'd never had harmful consequences—assuming that escaping a DUI is not one. This was about to change. It was budget season, and I was working on the hotel's next-year financial assumptions and the marketing plan on a Saturday morning when I began to feel my heartbeat fast immediately followed by numbness in my left arm. I kept working as the feelings were intensifying little by little. I decided to Google my symptoms and make sure that the numbness in my arm was not related to a possible heart attack. Big mistake. As I kept reading all the endless possibilities of my symptoms, my heart went crazy, and I began to lose my vision. I thought to myself, *This is it—I will die*. My entire life began to flash in my head, just a picture book rapidly turning pages. One of my coworkers was at the office, so I shouted out to her to call 911 because I was having a heart attack. I laid down on the floor hoping I would pass out and that it would make me feel better and avoid death. But I stayed conscious. The EMT team arrived and began to run tests on me. They concluded it was not a stroke or heart attack but a strong panic attack. My first of many.

Everyone at the hotel must have known the ambulance was there for me. I could see many of the associates watching as I was loaded in for an evaluation at the hospital. My boss and several co-workers sent me caring texts to ensure I was ok and resting once I returned home from the hospital. I blamed my breakdown on the stress of budget season when explaining the incident to my co-workers. However, I knew deep down that it had something to do with my drinking.

Thankfully I never had such a strong panic attack again, but I had many more which led me to get Xanax prescriptions. To fix issues related with one drug I began to take another one. The beauty of modern medicine—it is all about the quick fix versus finding the root cause of issues. As I began to feel more relaxed and normal, not suffering from anxiety or having too much trembling from damage to my nervous system, my alcoholic consumption continued to increase.

Powerful Lessons

- There's no such thing as a lucky day. If you escape a DUI, a divorce, or death (your own or someone else's), while continuing to abuse a substance or behavior, it's only a matter of time.
- When it comes to addiction, usually by the time someone begins to suspect that something might be wrong, chances are you are already in serious trouble.
- Addicts often want the consequences they are experiencing to change without changing their habits—the definition of insanity.

Chapter 3: A Party of One

Addiction is a very lonely disease. In San Antonio, I began to isolate and distance myself from others. The hospitality business always allows for a very social environment, and that holds true particularly for the sales team not only due to internal interactions but also because of the engagement with guests and customers and the entertaining that goes along with this. But as the disease progressed, those connections became mostly superficial ones. I had few close friends, which was something unimaginable for me. At that time, the real Cesar—the kind, warm-hearted, empathetic, and caring one—was gone. It was like my soul had been sucked out of me, and a vacuum was left inside. All I cared about was myself and how I could keep drinking as much as possible. Nothing more, nothing less.

Laura and I had distanced from each other a lot and we barely socialized with others because of the progression of my addiction. She knew things were not right. I believe she realized I was a changed person when I hosted a holiday office party for my team. Once the night was over, she told me that she never saw me so distant and without a bond with other people. It was like there was no chemistry among my team members and me, she said. That hurt me. One of my strongest suits and sources of pride I have is how much I care about people and that I can create deep and meaningful connections regardless of the background of a person. That is a big part of who I am, and that was gone; she knew it. I was not ready to admit it, however.

Biology: My Test Results

In March 2023, I received my Biomarker Evaluation Report with the custom panel results that identified, isolated, and measured specific biomarkers relating to my mental health. Not surprisingly, there were polymorphisms or SNPs (error in genetic coding) that can contribute to behaviors such as risk taking, impulse control, addiction, anxiety, and depression.

In simpler terms, the test results highlighted significant details about specific chemicals in my brain and body, including neurotransmitters (which are like messengers in the brain) and hormones. These chemicals include:

- Epinephrine and Norepinephrine: Often associated with the body's stress response, they are responsible for the "fight or flight" reaction, increasing heart rate and energy in stressful situations. An imbalance can lead to issues like anxiety, high blood pressure, heart palpitations, and sleep disturbances. Excess levels can cause chronic stress, while low levels can lead to a lack of focus and energy.
- Glutamate: This acts as the brain's main "on" switch, crucial for learning and memory. As a key neurotransmitter for cognitive functions, an excess of glutamate can overstimulate the brain,

potentially causing excitotoxicity, which is harmful to brain cells. This can contribute to neurological disorders. Low levels can lead to symptoms like fatigue, poor concentration, and mood disorders.
- Gamma-Aminobutyrate (GABA): Serving as the brain's "off" switch, it helps in calming the brain and reducing nerve activity. Low levels can lead to anxiety, chronic stress, and epilepsy. Excessive GABA activity can result in sedation and can affect cognitive functioning.
- Histamine: This is known for its role in allergies, but in the brain, it's involved in wakefulness. High levels can lead to allergies, sleep issues, and headaches, while low levels might result in fatigue, low stomach acid, and susceptibility to viral infections.
- Phenethylamine: Found naturally in the body and in foods like chocolate, it's linked to mood regulation. Low levels are associated with depression and attention deficit disorders, while high levels might contribute to schizophrenia.
- DHEA: A "parent" hormone that can transform into other hormones, impacting mood and health. Low levels are associated with aging, fatigue, muscle loss, and decreased bone density. High levels can lead to hormonal imbalances, including those that affect mood.
- Cortisol: This stress hormone has a daily rhythm, peaking in the morning and decreasing throughout

the day, influencing mood and fear. High levels can lead to weight gain, high blood pressure, sleep disturbances, and a weakened immune system. Low levels can result in chronic fatigue, low blood pressure, and mood disorders.

While these terms may seem complex, the essential point is clear: the way these chemicals and hormones behave and interact has a profound connection to my actions and feelings, particularly concerning my addiction experiences. The balance and levels of these substances in my body significantly influence my behavioral patterns and the challenges I face with addiction. This understanding provides a more nuanced view of the biochemical factors contributing to my addictive behaviors reducing the enigma of my journey by quite a bit. When I had my first call with Dr. Higgins to review the above results, which was supported by a very robust report, I was overwhelmed and a bit shocked, to say the least. The initial shock subsidized quite a bit as we agreed on the plan to treat my chemical imbalances and the reassurance that she would be alongside me in the next six months to ensure our plan was working and my chemicals were improving as expected.

Environment: The Shadow of Rebellion

After my mother died when I was 12, I was very afraid of being attached to someone or something. As a result, I always abruptly cut off a relationship or ties for no other reason other than fear of being hurt and feeling pain. I felt

I would rather be the one hurting than the one being hurt. Upon reflection, this affected my relationship with my father, my brother, my stepmom, close friends and even at some of my jobs. It felt good when I was the one in control and decided when something ended. By doing so, I never had to be afraid of getting hurt again because if I felt as if there was the slightest inclination that an end may be nearing, I would just pull the plug. When I experienced my mom's death, I learned firsthand that life is not fair, and it can hurt. I did not know this at the time but by practicing this behavior, it was the start of my selfishness and self-centeredness and slowly I was becoming my "own God." I felt I could control things and outcomes.

As part of my coping journey with the loss of my mom, I began to project normalcy in my life. It was much easier to present a happy front where I did not have to experience and confront the painful feelings I had of fear, sadness anger and loneliness. My approach was made easier because at home, we never spoke about our feelings or what was happening deep within us. Like the journey of becoming my "own God," this smoke-and-mirrors lifestyle helped me develop some very important social skills. While it has cost me dearly in the long run, it allowed for short term gains in my personal and professional life. Though some short cuts can seem effective at first, it certainly wasn't in my case as it prevented me from knowing how to deal with my emotions and learning that not being perfect or having bad days is completely acceptable.

As you can imagine our life in Brazil did not improve after my mom's passing. I can't speak for all my family but to me those next few years were very painful ones. Thankfully I had my school and "street" friends to help me escape reality, and while it helped me being around them, looking back I could see the progression in my rebellion— in all areas of my life. It became a shadow that was always following me.

Throughout the next few years, I developed a fantastic ability to charm myself out of tough situations and get my way since I was able to easily connect with people and put up a front when needed. I had a keen ability to read people, knew what they wanted to hear and what their weaknesses were, so I preyed on them to get what I wanted. I am not proud to admit this, but I became a very good manipulator. One lighthearted example is when I was in college in Switzerland and had an English exam. Later, I will share more about my experience in college, but for now just picture that I am in a foreign country studying in a language that I had very basic understanding at most. I wrote all the answers to the best of my ability, but my handwriting can be hard to read. At times I cannot even read it 😊. My English professor was unable to read the exam. He was a very nice man and asked me to go to his office to review the test with him. As he was reading the questions and sharing his understanding of my written answers, I would share just enough information based on the hints he was giving me so that I could influence his

52

interpretation of what I wrote versus what I meant. I ended up getting a C+ instead of what was most likely a F.

While there are many innocent and funny moments in my life such as the one above, this way of living created a façade where people saw the happy, super friendly, caring Cesar even though there was a lot of pain and turmoil happening inside me. Because I ignored this issue most of my life, the compounded effect of bottling it up for many years, ended up having distraught consequences not only for me but to the ones closest to me.

Development: Addiction Over Education

As I mentioned, my father gave a lot of importance to our studies. So, if I had acceptable grades (at least 6.5 out of 10, or a passing grade when I studied in Brazil), I was free to go out with my friends. In his view I had earned the right to do whatever I wanted since I was responsible enough to meet the minimum grade requirements at school. Little did he know that my average grades were not achieved through hard work but due to my cheating expertise. I worked very hard on my plots to cheat, influence teachers, and copy exams from previous years so that my freedom was not disrupted.

I was free to let myself loose. Going to clubs and bars when I was 13 and 14 became a frequent occurrence, and the drinking evolved from beer to hard liquor and mixed drinks. The high I got from drinking was like no other feeling I had experienced in my life. There was nothing to worry about; nothing could bring me down—I was invincible and the life of the party.

Clearly you don't have to be a M.D or a psychic to know that my early and frequent encounters with alcohol were more than a perfect "training ground" for my addiction. I would never shy away from it and from what I can recall, there was nothing else I was as committed as I was to my partying and drinking.

I know that many addicts have had different paths and experiences. This is the scary side of this illness. Many addicts I have met are not aware of any addicts in their family, had no known trauma or did not start to drink early in their lives. There is no certain path to be or to become an addict. This is one of the reasons why addiction is so dangerous and easily misunderstood. Everyone is different and every path is different, but all of them will have the same result unless something is done about it—death. It is that simple. I came close to it a few times even when I thought it was under control.

Denial and Justification

Addiction truly distorts your thinking, your views, and your feelings. Instead of having a natural reaction of self-reflection and taking a deep look into myself and what was happening to me after Laura brought her observations to my attention in 2011 after my team holiday party. I rejected these observations as she clearly had no idea what she was talking about, and she was in no place to judge the connection I have with my team. It was a different team than the ones I had before therefore a different dynamic. My defense mechanism was complete denial and justification of anything and everything that seemed off to her or anyone else.

Close to the end of our two years in San Antonio, Laura and I were almost strangers. We were so far apart from each other. I was in a sick state of mind, drunk all the time, giving her plenty of reasons and opportunities to pull away from me. I cannot imagine the pain and confusion I caused her. I was ruining our lives and her trust in me.

Once the end of my two-year contract was approaching, I made the decision to request a transfer. It was my only hope. Of course, as I reasoned, all the issues I had, and the horrible disintegration of our marriage had nothing to do with my drinking or myself but instead it was all work related. Remember, I was always hunting for happiness on the outside versus from within.

I was very fortunate to have the support from my boss and the regional sales vice president therefore my request to relocate was quickly granted. The transfer took us to Fort Lauderdale, Florida. Now I thought to myself, *We will have a fresh start and everything will be different*. Sound familiar?

It was June 2013, and we were living in Fort Lauderdale. Everything was exciting, we were super happy, we were living in this huge condo at the hotel I had just relocated. It was gorgeous and right in front of the beach—life was great! Or was it?

Living at the hotel provided me with great and easy access to alcohol whenever I wanted. There was plenty of beer and wine in the condo, I could sign off on whatever I wanted at the hotel bars, and I found a liquor store close by that sold some cheap vodka in addition to the "10% local discount" I qualified for. This set-up allowed me to use spare cash to buy liquor and fly under Laura's radar as I did not use any of our debit or credit cards, which would have caused her to question any suspicious charges, especially if there was any possible correlation with alcohol.

My habits from San Antonio just intensified. I was drinking non-stop, even beer or whatever I could get my hands on during work hours; I did not care about the possibility of someone smelling my beer breath. I was going into the hotel guestrooms, which had large liquor minibar bottles—a quarter of a traditional bottle—unlike the typical small liquor bottles seen in most hotel minibars. But these bottles had tricky safety seals which would have been impossible for me to reseal, so I turned away from my usual go to (vodka) to the half-bottles of wine. I'd have one or two of them in one room, and as I felt no buzz, I'd repeat the process in another guestroom until it got the job done. It was madness! After chugging the contents of those bottles, I would refill them with water. Thanks to the dark glass of the red wine bottles and the green tint of the white wine ones, it was impossible to tell what liquid they contained just by looking. This illusion remained intact until someone opened a bottle to drink from it. I was very good at resealing the screw caps. By carefully aligning the ridges of the cap with the metal skirt on the bottle's neck, I made sure they appeared untampered with—a scary trait to have mastered.

After living a few months at the hotel condo, we found our house. As we got settled into our new house in Fort Lauderdale, my morning routine on my way to work became stopping by Publix every morning to get two to three boxes of wine. Instead of the bottles I used to buy in San Antonio, I "upgraded" to box wine as the packaging was easier to hide in the car and to eventually discard without calling too much attention to myself. Also, I was no longer buying red wine for my breakfast. Instead, I opted for white wine just in case there was a little spill on my clothes while I drove and drank. I'd had some close calls with red wine in San Antonio and in the hotel guestrooms since arriving in Fort Lauderdale, so why risk getting red wine stains on my work clothes while driving to work? At the time this thought process was reasonable to me and I was actually proud of it as it was pretty clever, and I was getting away with it. Very sad! The only safety I was worried about was not having a stain on my clothes instead of the possibility of killing someone or myself while drinking and driving.

As I always used to go to the same Publix on my way to work and get the wine, as much as I wanted to avoid conversing with the cashier, it would happen from time to time. I recall one day she asked me if I had any plans with the boxes I was buying and I mentioned that it was for dinner since we had a big family at home. She began to tell me a story about a lady that used to buy a small box of wine and go straight to their bathroom to drink it. I told her that the lady must have some serious issues even though I was having three times the volume this bathroom lady was having.

In my view, I still had it under control because I was *choosing* to drink not because I *had* to drink. However, by now, I was drinking in the morning to stop the trembling and get out of the misery I was feeling from barely having any quality sleep. As a matter of fact, I recall vividly waking up one day around 3am and having to go to the kitchen and chug a few beers down to stop my hands tremor. Amazingly enough, in my mind I still did not have an issue; I was able to justify it in my mind and make sense out of it. I was leaving in an alternate reality.

Another method I mastered to purchase alcohol without Laura being aware was to stop at gas stations. I would go inside, ask the cashier to open my pump, and then I would pump some gas and go back inside to buy some beer, wine and sometimes those spiced-up lemonades, since they had less of an odor. The cashier would ring up everything to fit in one charge, which would usually equal about a full tank of gas. There was no way Laura could ever even imagine such a scenario, almost no person ever would—no person in their right mind would ever think of such scenario and I was confident she would never challenge a gasoline bill. After all, my Jeep was not economical, so I had the perfect excuse in case she ever questioned the frequency of gas charges.

As my drinking intensified so did my reasoning to sustain it. There was always a reason to drink. If I had a good day I needed to celebrate, if I had a stressful day at work, I had to forget it, if someone made me mad, I had to get back at them by drinking, and if I had an important meeting I had to drink to feel as if I was 10 feet tall and invincible. The danger of escalation in addiction is that the longer you get away with it, the more entitled you feel of doing what you are doing. After all, if I never had any major consequence happening to me, why should I change? I got away from a DUI, I overcame panic attacks with Xanax, I was one of the sales rising stars of the company and constantly got raving reviews on how great I was doing even though I was always hammered. In my sick mind, other than my nagging wife who was frequently suspicious of me, no one else seemed to have a problem with how I was carrying my life including myself.

By this time Laura was pretty much done with me. In San Antonio, we had grown apart and I think she did not have much time to digest and interpret what was going on with us as Gabby was just a baby and in need of her 24/7. As time passed by, Gabby was getting a bit more self-sufficient, allowing Laura to have some time for herself and consequently more time to realize the new Cesar and how disgusted she was by him. I had always lied about my drinking, and I was lying more and more about it; telling the truth was becoming the exception for me. I was always very defensive when questioned and tried to manipulate the situation by turning it around. This was not working any more. She knew better.

I became a hyper self-centered person with no regard to anyone. Laura lost all trust she had in me and rightfully so. It was easy to see and feel the deception she was feeling. She could not comprehend what was going on with the love of her life. This Cesar was not the Cesar she knew and married. *What happened to him? What went wrong, and how did he get to this point?*

This went on for a while until May 2014, just shy of a year since moving to Fort Lauderdale. At some point I brought up to Laura that our relationship was clearly not the same and that we should stop fooling ourselves. How grown up and mature of me. I was happy to discuss anything that was not related to my drinking even though it was the cause of all our issues. Was it worth considering a divorce? Should we go to a psychologist? We both agreed that we were disconnected, and that we should give ourselves a shot at finding the love and passion we used to have for one another.

We began going to a therapist. Our first session was a good step towards our goal but not super helpful. I began opening up about our issues except for the main one—my drinking. Of course, in my view it was mostly Laura's fault. I recall saying that I did not see the sparkle on her eyes anymore. Poor Cesar, how dare she not jump up and down when I walked through the door acting like a zombie?

When it was Laura's turn to speak, she mentioned that what hurt her the most was my drinking and the impact it was having on me and consequently on us. As a reminder, she did not know a tenth of what I was drinking, but the little glimpse of chaos she saw and the times she caught me in a lie had already had a tremendous effect on her, our relationship, and my behavior as a husband/father. Needless to say, I was not the same guy she married.

That resonated with me. I love my wife and did not want to hurt her. I wanted her to be happy, and be proud of who I was, and I deeply missed our connection and our happiness as a couple. Of course, I did not open up about my drinking, but I convinced Laura and myself that I saw her point and would be better with my drinking; I would be able to control it. I realized I needed to be there for her as the insecurity I was causing her was devastating.

I tried. We agreed just to drink on the weekends. I went a few days without drinking, but it did not last. I began sneaking alcohol once again and defaulting to my old habits. I was stopping by Publix to get my wine for breakfast, buying vodka to get me going throughout the day and then preparing myself mentally to act normal and sober once I got home so Laura would not know I had been drinking.

Of course, I always had some alcohol in my car, so I could sneak out to the garage whenever I had the opportunity and chug it down to keep my high. A lot of times I would place the drinks (either a bottle of vodka or wine) under the step tire in the trunk so that no one would ever find it. Even though we had recently chatted about how much my drinking bothered her, if I was high, life was great. All the worries would go away, I felt happy, and no one could bring me down—I was in my own little world, and it was the best place to be. I felt I could act to meet and fulfill her needs versus staying true to my word and my commitment to her.

And so, this kept going for almost two months. We went to therapy, I put on the show of my life pretending to be this great guy, saying everything I knew the therapist wanted to hear to gain her support and not get cornered on my issues. I did everything I could to ensure my habits were never brought up, so I could continue to drink. Deflection was very effective to accomplish this goal.

But at some point, my "lucky" streak would have to come to a halt. One day Laura had a hair appointment and needed me to get back from work a bit early so I could take care of Gabby. I arrived a few minutes late, and Laura was standing outside with Gabby. She was anxious to make it to her appointment on time. As Laura was handing

Gabby over to me, I could tell she knew I was hammered. She said: "Seriously? The one time I ask you to be there for me this is what happens?"

That was it.

The next day I knew I had to do something. I told Laura that I would handle my drinking once and for all. I decided to stop drinking. I stopped for 30 days. During the 30 days I truly had nothing to drink. I began to feel better and slowly began to romanticize the idea that I I may not have a drinking problem since I was able to stop.

Since my mid 20s I have taken medicine for cholesterol and high blood pressure. So, in 2014 as this was happening, I went to my doctor for a regular physical and cholesterol check. I was about 30 days sober, so I assumed my cholesterol had drastically dropped even though I had decided to stop taking my pills.

My results were in, and they were not what I was hoping for. My cholesterol was higher than the previous reading and it was gut wrenching. I thought to myself, *Even though I stopped drinking for 30 days, there has been no improvement to my cholesterol levels, so why keep my "healthy" lifestyle going? If I will be unhealthy anyways, I would rather be unhealthy and drunk.*

As you may recall, one of the fuels for my addiction was how poorly I handled my emotions, and it was back in full force. Self-pity was my default and comfort zone to justify some of my drinking and my "unfair" mentality. Poor

Cesar: my cholesterol wasn't good therefore life sucked; it wasn't worth living. At the time, this was the perfect excuse for self-pity to overtake my feelings and thoughts and once again give me the justification I needed to go back to drinking.

Powerful Lessons

- Addicts can easily create a façade where people see the happy, super friendly, caring outside when there is a lot of pain and turmoil happening inside. Ignoring this issue can cause long-term distress for not only the addicts but also those close to them.
- The danger of escalation in addiction is that the longer you get away with it, the more entitled you feel of doing what you are doing.
- If addicts are high, life can be great. All the worries go away—we feel happy, and no one can bring us down—we are in our own little worlds, and it is the best place to be.

Chapter 4: The Wake-Up Call

In July 2014, the day I received my cholesterol results coincided with one of my relapses. A few weeks earlier, I had planned a team meeting followed by a go-karting outing, which was set to happen that day. As soon as I decided to relapse, I reverted to my old habits and stopped by Publix to purchase three of my favorite wines en route to the team meeting. I consumed one bottle in roughly 10 minutes just before my arrival. We had the meeting, and afterwards, as we made our way to the go-kart facility, I felt a mix of emotions: half excitement for the upcoming activity and half frustration with the world over the "shocking" cholesterol results.

As I parked my car at the go-kart place, I drank a half bottle prior to walking in to make sure I would stay high. As we began our laps, I was driving like a maniac, bumping everyone out of my way thinking that I was Michael Schumacher. I was especially proud that I got the fastest lap of the team, and I was hammered. *How great was I?* In between drives I went to my car and drank more and more. Suddenly it hit me hard. I began to slur my speech and could barely stand up. Everyone quickly noticed and began to express their concern about me. *What was going on with Cesar?*

Since there was no alcohol being served at the facility, nobody seemed to suspect I'd been drinking. I recall being questioned about what was going on and I wasn't sure what to say. *What could I possibly say to justify my state?* That was until someone asked me if I was having a heat stroke. There—I had the perfect excuse. I jumped all over it as it was very hot (summer in south Florida) and something like that could be very plausible given we were in a hot facility driving go-karts. This way, no one would know about my drinking habit. You see, as usual, everything works out for Cesar. I told my team that I would wait a bit and then just drive home. But not so fast, as they had already called the EMT and Laura.

The ambulance arrived. The paramedics began to run my vitals inside the ambulance and soon realized everything was pretty good—there was nothing wrong with me. They asked me what was going on. I told them not to tell anyone, but I was just drunk. While I was in the ambulance, taking the test and talking to the medics, some fantastic people from my team were helping my wife. They were keeping her posted on what was going on and that I was ok. Laura was really puzzled as to what could be possibly happening and told one of my teammates that it could have been alcohol and to check my car for it. They checked my car and found my wine boxes in the center console and under the seat. My façade had finally crumbled, there was no more justifying my actions, behavior or giving a plausible excuse about having three empty boxes of wine in the car. Laura arrived to pick me up and brought me home. I saw her and my beautiful daughter Gabby and I was distraught. I felt complete defeat and shame.

That was my wake-up call! The next morning, I decided that I was done with my double life. I was tired of being dishonest with myself and wanted to feel good and proud of who I was once again. Furthermore, I was determined to spare my daughter the pain, fear, and anger that I experienced growing up. These feelings from being around my father's drinking habits were still very real. Passing on those feelings to her was the last thing I wanted Gabby to experience. I still had time to turn things around and ensure she didn't have to endure the same feelings I did growing up. By breaking this painful and vicious cycle, I wanted to give her the chance to feel loved, cared for, and safe. I also would love for her to experience a trusting and close relationship with her father. Ultimately, it was up to me to provide that opportunity.

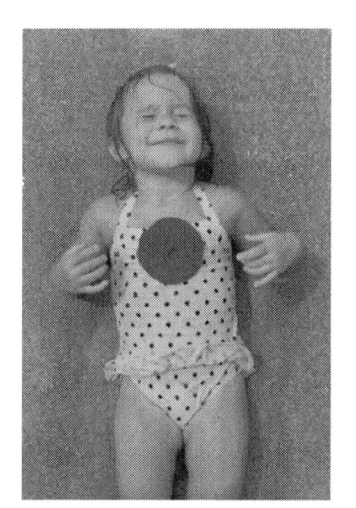

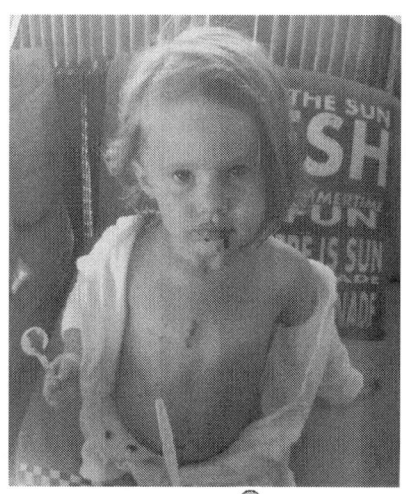

Gabby as a toddler in Florida...the cutest thing ever 😊

Biology: Genetic Coding

In 2023, while researching the biology behind my addiction, I was perhaps too caught up in the euphoria and pride of being eight years sober. This led me to believe that everything was "perfect:" I thought that since I wasn't drinking or craving alcohol, there was no further work needed on the addiction front. However, my call with Dr. Higgins left me feeling partly relieved to learn more about the science of addiction, but also partly overwhelmed by the extent of work still required to optimize my mental health. As we reviewed my results, I started to grasp the complexity of addiction. It was particularly enlightening when Dr. Higgins explained that there were several SNPs (genetic coding errors) that are highly correlated with my genetic predisposition to addiction, including MAO-B, GAD 1, HTR2, CoQ2, among others. MAO-B, GAD1, HTR2A, and CoQ2 are all genes that are involved in various biological processes in the body, and I had never heard of any of them before, so I did some reading to understand what each of them meant to further digest the information and conversation I just had with Dr. Higgins.

- MAO-B (Monoamine oxidase B) is an enzyme that breaks down neurotransmitters like dopamine, norepinephrine, and serotonin in the brain. Genetic variations in the MAO-B gene have been linked to an increased risk of Parkinson's disease, depression, and aggression. I have not had any official diagnosis of any of these risks, however I can have mood swings, especially when I get very hungry or "hangry" 😊

- GAD1 (Glutamic acid decarboxylase 1) is an enzyme that is involved in the synthesis of the neurotransmitter GABA. GABA is a chemical serving as the brain's "off" switch; it helps calm the brain and reduce nerve activity. Low levels can lead to anxiety, which I had a history of as well as difficulty sleeping.
- HTR2A (Serotonin receptor 2A) is a receptor protein that binds to the neurotransmitter serotonin. Serotonin is a chemical that carries messages between nerve cells in the brain and throughout your body. Serotonin plays a key role in such body functions as mood, sleep, digestion, nausea, bone health, and wound healing, among others. Genetic variations in the HTR2A gene have been linked to an increased risk of mental disorders such as depression, anxiety, and bipolar disorder.

CoQ2 (Coenzyme Q10 biosynthesis protein 2) is an enzyme that is involved in the production of CoQ10, a molecule that plays a role in cellular energy production. CoQ10 is a powerful antioxidant substance that helps convert food into energy. Basically, if you have a mitochondrial disease, your cells can't produce enough energy. I was very surprised by this result as I consider myself having a fair amount of energy and can do a lot of activities (work and non-work) throughout the day. It showed me how much I was just pushing through out of sheer willpower. While there isn't a cure, it was part of the treatment that Dr. Higgins proposed for the next few months.

These were some of the areas that I have been working with Dr. Higgins throughout our virtual appointments. It has been great to feel a difference in my mind and body after going through the program.

Environment: Studying in São Paulo

When I was 18, I was the life of the party, and I had my drinking under control.

Or so I thought. For any non-addict I was way out of control during this part of my life. But in my mind, this was a timeframe that even though my drinking was clearly excessive I still did not feel dependency and the need to have a drink to function. Basically, the drinking was not having negative effects on my health and on my life even though I was on my path to addiction.

Up to that point I had never been a very disciplined person in most areas of my life except for "having a good time" or any activity that would involve drinking. From my days as a young adolescent, no matter what the environment was, I always felt as if I belonged as long as there was alcohol.

College, I believe, had a strong influence on my eventual addiction. My first year of college I was still in São Paulo. Throughout my school life I never had good grades. Most of my classes prior to college had around 30 to 40 students and I was always on the bottom six or so. When it came time to decide what path I would take to college, it was not like I had many options. Law, medicine, or engineering were never in the cards for me. In Brazil, GPA has no bearing whatsoever on getting into a college or university, but you have to go through different phases of tests where you directly compete with other students going for those same courses—I had no chance on any of the highly coveted courses or at the top universities. As such, when selecting colleges, I defaulted to a degree where I could use my social skills to get a diploma. I reasoned this would allow me to check off the college box for my dad, not feel like a complete loser and hopefully feel some level of accomplishment. Hospitality was a major relatively young in the late 90s, so it was a perfect choice for me, as any warm body would be able to understand it.

My hotel school in São Paulo was relaxed and my classes were in the evening, but I spent most of my first year in college not attending college. There was a little "boteco" (bar) on the corner of the block, so I hung out there with the "cool" people. Attending classes was a rare event.

Along with "studying," I got a job in the hotel industry to complement my technical knowledge with practical experience. I will never forget that day. I was so proud that I got a job; it was a new 5-star hotel in São Paulo and a pretty coveted workplace, so it was fairly difficult to be hired—it was a rigorous process. Even though I applied to be a room service busboy earning 500 dollars a month, some basic skills of English were required. I barely qualified, so it felt like hitting the lottery, and I was very proud of my achievement.

Life was good! Instead of attending class I had a great time drinking beer, eating, and chatting all night long before I headed to work for my overnight shift as a room service busboy.

Funny thing, at work—where most people begin to grow and develop into a responsible person—I began to learn more tricks toward my addiction journey. First day at work: 11pm on a weekday. I had the graveyard shift. I showed up with plenty of time to get dressed in my nice uniform and begin my career journey. Unlike most days, I actually went to school immediately before heading to work and did not join my usual friends at the boteco for beers; after all, I was going to begin my career and had to be at my best. I walked into the room service area where we were stationed, and I was greeted by two professional waiters who were going to be my trainers and show me what the job is all about. They were two great guys, one in his mid-30s and one in his early 40s. My training began with a tour of the area so that I could get familiarized with my surroundings and be able to perform all duties from prepping a delivery tray and cart to cleaning and disposing of dirty dishes. The first area they showed me was a huge ice machine. They showed me where the buckets were and the location of the ice scoop, and then they opened the ice machine. What was inside? Ice of course, with a bunch of beer in it. And not just any beer. It was a very good national beer called Cerpa which was difficult to find and was a perfect match to our five-star surroundings.

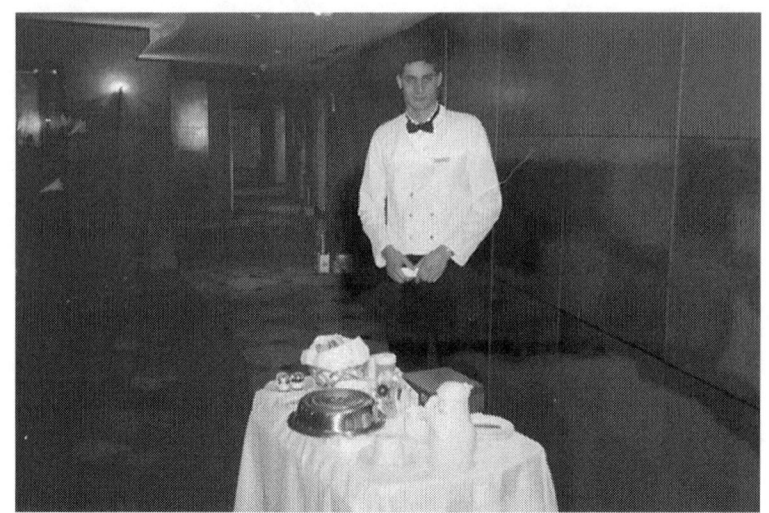

Delivering breakfast - probably drunk.

Development: The Beginning of My Career

While I was excited about the prospect of having beers at work, I was quite uneasy. This was a dream job and the beginning of my career—I could not screw it up on Day 1. Were these waiters showing me the beer as a test put in place by management to make sure I would not break any policies and procedures? Or was it a nice warm welcome for the new kid? Neither, I soon discovered. It was a way to ensure that I was going to be "in the system" and not disrupt their day-to-day in any way, shape, or form. By including me on it in my first night, they quickly established how things were run, and that I was part of it. I was part of the system, and I was one of them. I could not report their behavior or opt out of the system.

And so, it began—drinking almost every day at the boteco and at work.

I worked at the hotel for about 9 months, during which time our drinking spilled beyond our secret "office" area. We began drinking on guest-room floors as well. Every night we had to collect the trays that had been delivered earlier in the day. Most of them were placed in the hallways, but there were quite a few dirty trays left in checked-out rooms, and these were our favorites. As overachievers, we took not only the trays out of the rooms but also some minibar souvenirs. Our drink of choice was a Rusty Nail (Drambuie and Scotch); I did not know the name of this cocktail at the time but came to enjoy it immediately. The building was more than 20 floors tall, and we typically had drinks every couple of floors. The drinking did not stop there. Once we brought all dirty trays down to our area, we would begin to separate the dishes, glasses, etc., and we always ensured that no alcohol left over by guests was wasted, whether it was flat, warm Champagne or leftover wine bottles.

About 6 months into the job, I got a call from my dad. He asked me how I would feel about continuing my education in Switzerland. He did some research, as he was always concerned with education, and found a great option for a best-in-class degree. I was ecstatic! Besides the images of a prolonged vacation coming through my mind it was great timing because the first year of college was soon coming to an end, and I was tanking in most of my classes, either by lack of attendance or simply poor scores. His offer to make Switzerland possible was that he would pay for tuition, and I would cover my living expenses. I did not hesitate a minute and we had a deal.

I was very happy to have this awesome opportunity ahead of me. Besides the fact that I was heading to a great place to explore and party, I was going to start my school fresh and not have to face any consequences for messing around during my first school year. But not so fast! One little detail my dad shared a few weeks after we agreed on the opportunity in Switzerland was that I would need my college transcripts to get credit for all my courses taken in São Paulo.

I was freaking out. How would I tell him that I had nothing to show for my year in college and that I would not be able to get any credit? This could not happen—my dream to go to Switzerland would be over.

Since I needed to quickly figure out a way to salvage this opportunity, my manipulation skills, the skills that go hand in hand with alcoholism, kicked in. This was the perfect opportunity for me to put these skills to use; after all, I really needed the transcripts as all our financial assumptions for me to go to Switzerland were based on getting full credit from my first year in college. I don't recall how many courses I was taking in my first year, but it was quite a few. I do recall at least 3 to 4 in which I was in serious trouble and would not pass unless there was a small miracle.

After some thought, I approached the director of the hotel school in São Paulo and explained the situation to her. Despite my best efforts I was having challenges with the aggressive and intense curriculum at this great institution, and that it would be very helpful if she could assist me in any way to get my grades to a passing score so that the Swiss option could remain viable. But wait, what about my poor attendance? Well, I told her that it was because of my work commitment, and all the extra shifts I had proactively taken whenever possible to further complement my studies with practical experience—which of course was a complete lie.

The true reason for my poor attendance, as you know, was my frequent drinking escapades. One of the key selling points for non-Ivy League schools is their students' high employability rates, which they use to attract more students. I was aware that this wouldn't alter my past attendance record, but I believed it could serve as a strong argument for the director to consider. Additionally, I assured her that moving forward, I was fully committed to my studies and would not miss any more classes. The director, who was a very kind person, encouraged me to focus and dedicate myself to studying. She promised to consider possible solutions in the meantime.

So there I was, half relieved that there was a chance I wouldn't have to come clean to my dad on how I was wasting his tuition money and half-frustrated that I could not continue with my bar activity during my classes; but thankfully because of my job I did not have to worry about it as I had an 8-hour window of opportunity for plenty of drinking with my co-workers.

During the last two months of my first year in college I applied myself to improve my scores, but mostly by cheating on tests as well as manipulating results. I recall altering the IT teacher's grading master sheet by accessing his file during a class break. There were 5 projects in total for the year and all of mine were unchecked as I had not completed any of them. During one of the classes breaks he left the grading sheet unattended on his desk and I took the opportunity to alter the grades by marking that I had completed four out of the five IT projects. My commitment to attendance and my cheating, in addition to some possible help from the director, ensured I passed all my classes. While they were not great scores, they were enough to get me out of trouble at home and begin my studies in Switzerland.

Drinking Like a Fish and Partying Like a Rockstar

In January 1999 I arrived in Switzerland. What a beautiful country! While I had been in Europe a few times since my father was from Germany, it felt different. The scenic views of its beautiful lakes and mountains, to the beautiful, charming city in which I was going to live—it was almost surreal. Immediately after arriving in Brig by train from Zurich, I headed to my college to check-in, learn about my schedule and get instructions for the college dorm and other necessities of campus life.

The school curriculum was in English, and I barely knew any despite having taken English lessons back home for several years. One of the first things I did was to attend the orientation day, which was mandatory for all students. My English was so poor that when the director of my college began to share information on policies and procedures, I began to wonder after a few minutes into his presentation, *Why in the hell does this guy keep talking about the police?* 😊 Little did I know the difference between "policy" and "police." So go figure, studying had never been my forte, and now I suffered very poor handling of the language in which I would be studying. Now, I realized, I really had to step up my connections, so I could maneuver my way through courses, sharpen my cheating skills and most importantly make a lot of friends with the "cool guys"—the ones that had the same values as I did, to drink like a fish and party like a rockstar.

During my two years in Switzerland, my drinking began to get heavier and heavier. It started as a great social experience to get to know people and hangout at the pubs and the frequent house parties. It quickly escalated as of one of my jobs was bartending at one of the student bars with plenty of self-serving pours, and eventually grew into morning drinking on the weekends to keep the party going. I believe this was one of the turning points for me and my alcoholic journey. Up to that point even though I was drinking pretty much daily and for long periods of time, I always drank at acceptable drinking times by society standards. I'd drink in the afternoon or early evenings throughout the night or around brunch time on weekends—but never before breakfast or having a drink as my breakfast. Scary.

Throughout my time in Switzerland, I had different roommates. One of them was very sweet. His name was Stale, a Norwegian kid who became a dear friend. The way we became roommates was a bit unorthodox as I barely knew him up to that point. Stale struggled a lot with drugs (all kinds) and alcohol as well and the school was trying to help him get settled and socialize a bit more in hopes to make connections with other students and help him to do fewer drugs. I happily agreed to become roommates as I could see that he was a good guy. He was reserved but a person with a big heart.

Once we moved in, we spent a considerable amount of time together, but we never really hung out that often as I was not that much into drugs. The only drug I enjoyed was cocaine, but it was very expensive, and I hated the feeling of coming down from the high; it made me depressed, and I felt miserable—I am very thankful now that this was the case—otherwise instead of alcohol addiction, I would have had a much heavier one. Even though Stale and I did not spend a lot of time partying together it was easy to see how out of control he was. I recall seeing him one day in our room getting out of bed around 8am, crawling to the mini fridge in our dorm and drinking straight from the bottle of vodka along with about 10 sleeping pills. I thought to myself, *this is insane; this guy has a serious problem. I cannot even attempt to comprehend how someone would ever get to this point...who would want to be like this?*

There was a clear disparity in how we used our drugs of choice, but I was so oblivious or naïve, as I thought I was different. The best way I can describe it is when you see someone doing an action that is wrong but that you also do it, however you can justify your motives to yourself and delineate that you are doing for a different reason or what you are doing is not as bad as the other person. At that point, I believed I just drank to have fun and that it was always under control. I would never get to that point as I had just witnessed with Stale, or so I thought. In my mind, he was out of control for sipping straight vodka at 8am but having a case of beer early on the weekends at my friend's dorm listening to Andrea Bocelli and chatting until it was time to *really* start drinking was justifiable and acceptable to me. In my mind, I was in no way shape or form remotely like Stale as it related to substance abuse. My behavior and what I did was normal while his actions were not; so much so that I was one of the main influences on one of his stints in rehab. It was impressive how I could be so convincing to him and demonstrate that he had a problem and needed help while I was doing the same thing, just in a different format.

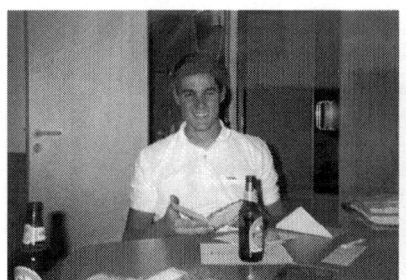

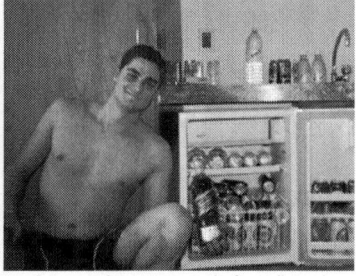

A weekend morning at the college dorm drinking beer and getting ready for a "good time" during a vacation visiting my family in Brazil.

Anything and everything I did with very few exceptions was surrounded by or included alcohol, from studying all night long for exams with an open bar to binging all night long at pubs and parties.

One great example of the intensity of my drinking was when a couple of friends of mine stopped by my dorm around midnight or so on a Friday asking me if I wanted to join them and head out to Sion (a city in Switzerland about an hour drive from Brig). They were heading to Sion because the decision for the 2006 Winter Olympic Games was going to be announced on Saturday. Sion and Turin were the finalist host cities so there was a huge party to be had. I wasn't in the mood but eventually agreed to it and took with me a couple of bottles of vermouth I had in my closet. To this day I have no idea how we made it to Sion as we drank a lot along the way. I vividly remember flashbacks of our group partying in the city with the locals. We were all eagerly awaiting the announcement the next day, thoroughly enjoying ourselves with lots more drinking and having a blast. Suddenly everything stopped, people were quiet, and you could hear a pin drop. This was because Sion lost the bid to Turin for the 2006 Winter Olympic Games, I found out later. People must have thought that we were the rudest people on earth as we carried on our partying as everyone stared in disbelief of another loss for Sion as a possible Winter Olympics host. I do, however, recall the drive back, during which all of us were still drunk, and the car weaving among the lanes as our friend who was driving was constantly falling asleep, and we kept waking him up to avoid a crash on our way home.

My college life went like this until graduation. Plenty of drinking without any consequences other than two hotel management diplomas despite having a very tough start with a 1.9 GPA in my first semester when I was threatened to be kicked out for six months by the school director. Somehow, I was able to complete my bachelor's degree in a three-year window through an accelerated program. My lucky streak continued; things always worked out even though I did not put forth the effort. There was never a consequence; so why should I change anything?

Upon graduation I was offered an internship at a hotel in Atlanta. How great! Quite a few students graduating from hotel school in Switzerland strive to get internships in the U.S., and after many interviews I got my opportunity. Besides the joy of having a career prospect and start building my adult life in the best possible way, I was very excited that I had just turned 21, therefore within the legal drinking age in the U.S.

But this time was different; I was serious about my job. I really wanted to achieve my goals of eventually becoming a hotel sales manager, so I was really dedicated to the work. I did not drink at the job but also did not change my habits outside of work. It was almost like I went back to my routine in high school. I'd get my stuff done during the day and then after that it was fair game—anything goes.

My efforts were paying off. I was quickly climbing the corporate ladder. Within four years I had been promoted from an intern to junior sales manager to national account manager (mid-level management). For most of those years I was going out from Wednesday to Sunday nights. That was my religion and wow, I was committed to it. To this day I still wonder how I could afford all those drinks as I was not making much money, did not have a credit card as I was building my credit score in the US, but somehow, I pulled it off. Perhaps the fact that I always got a buzz prior to going out may have made it financially feasible. I routinely blacked out, but because I was never a rowdy or an angry drunk, I never worried about doing something stupid. I would just hit on girls or stay friendly with people I just met. So, I had another great justification and reason not to change my habits. I'd think, *I am not quite sure what I did or what happened last night, but it could not have been that bad.*

At the time, the sales office I worked at was almost all men and most were single. It was a great environment for keeping my routine intact, and it supported my assumption that what I was doing was normal. Throughout the first four years of my career, I had no significant consequences, but I began to notice some warning signs and confirmation that my behavior was not normal. One example was when I showed up to work wearing the same clothes from the previous day. I'd partied non-stop from the time I left work until I showed up the following day. As we gathered for our daily stand-up meeting first thing in the morning, my boss noticed I was wearing the same clothes and sent me home for the day. In my mind, while I wasn't proud of being sent home, I justified my behavior as someone who was just having a good time.

Inseparable from Day One

St. Patrick's Day 2004. The day I met my soulmate, Laura. A mutual friend had introduced us, and it was love at first sight—at least for me. That was not the case with her. We had a great time, but she wanted to make sure that the time and connection we had was real and that it wasn't a one off or "too good to be true."

We spent the day together at Park Tavern, a bar and restaurant at Piedmont Park in Atlanta where we eventually got married a couple of year later. I got very drunk, as usual, and looking back it was another warning sign I should have caught on to the fact that my drinking was not normal. By the time I got back home I had lost two apartment keys—mine and my roommate's that he gave me after I lost my own. As I contemplated my options to call a locksmith or break into the apartment, I chose the latter. I end up breaking into my place through the front window with the empty vodka bottle that I had left on my deck from the previous night. It made complete sense at the time. *Why call and wait for a locksmith guy? Instead, get the vodka bottle and break the window to get into the apartment and pass out on my bed*. It certainly did not look like a great idea the next morning when I woke up and got a $130 quote for the glass replacement.

Laura and I were inseparable from Day One. I called her the next morning to check on her and say that I would love to see her again. We agreed to go to the movies that same day however there was a problem. My car was broken down (and I had no money to fix it). Once I shared this with Laura, I thought the date would be off and that I would be out of the picture. To my surprise she went along with it, and we ended up meeting at the movies—it was a weird movie with Johnny Depp, "The Secret Window." Despite the movie, we had a great time, and, on that day, I knew she was the one for me.

We immediately began dating seriously. Laura was an elementary school teacher and right after her summer vacation, during which she went to study Spanish in Peru, we moved in together. Or, to be more precise, I moved into her condo. Life was good and my drinking was not too bad during this time when comparing to my previous norm. I was drinking mostly in social situations (even though still heavy) but no major incidents or issues. Almost a year after living together I got a nice new job at another hotel in my first director role. At 25 years old I had surpassed my internal goal of having a sales director title by 27 or 28 and had this awesome woman by my side. Life was perfect!

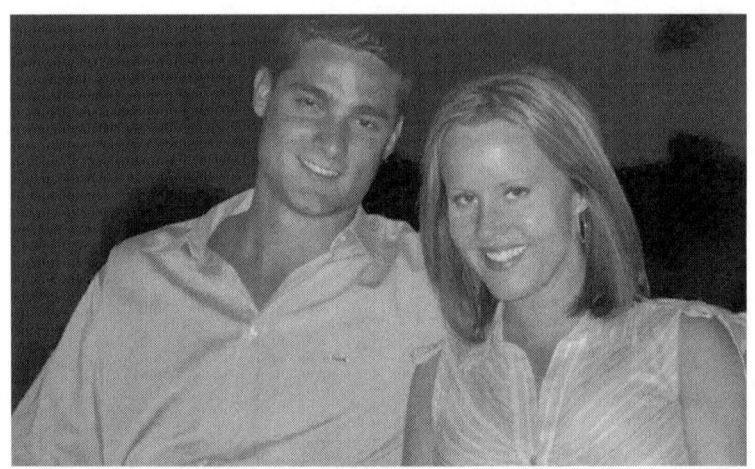

Me and Laura in the beginning of our relationship in 2004

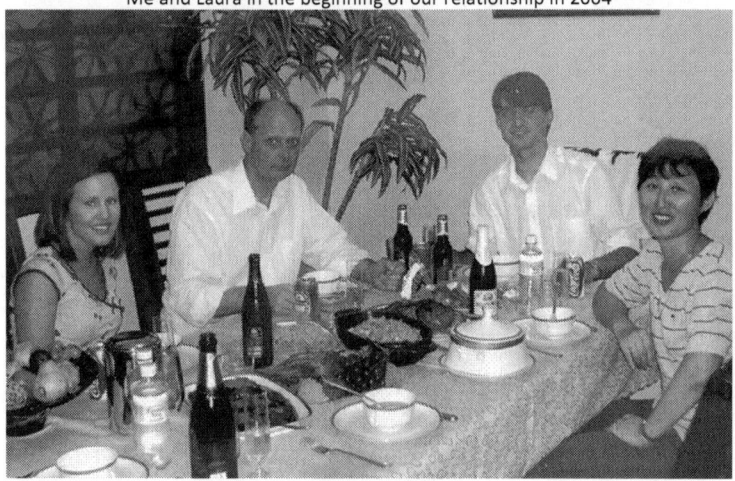

When Laura first met my family in December 2004. Laura, my dad, my brother, and Chong Hee. I proposed to her a few days later in Rio De Janeiro under a beautiful fireworks display on New Years.

Life was perfect until one of the customer receptions at my hotel a few months into the new job. We hosted several of our clients for a great outdoor evening function for appreciation and networking. I was drinking one of my favorite drinks, which was vodka soda. I must have had at least 10 to 12 drinks during the event and then of course as the bartender was breaking the bar down, I had to get my last double drink so I wouldn't sober up too fast, and I would have that nice buzz going for a while. I was having a great time.

Instead of calling Laura and asking her to pick me up from work, I did what I always did every time I was drunk. I drove. I got in my car and began to do my 5-mile commute. As I was leaving, I called Laura at home to give her assurance that I was okay and on my way home. I had all the windows down, so the car would not smell like a bar, however she could not hear me with all the background noise. She asked me to roll up the windows and she immediately realized I was under the influence. I assured her that I was ok and tried to hang up as fast as possible in hopes that my lie would stick. I ended the call with the following sentence, *"Don't worry baby; I am fine and will call you when I get home."* Moments later, I was pulled over by the police for the near-DUI.

Powerful Lessons

- Addicts can justify their behavior by comparing it to another's. One drinker, for example, might justify his motives as having fun while watching another drinker sip straight vodka at 8am. But if both have become powerless over alcohol, both are addicts, with the only certain outcome being eventual death.

- Enablers and codependents of addicts can come in all forms: friends at college, colleagues at work, spouses. This can be intentional or unintentional.
- When we are addicted, our thoughts and actions become insane as we often believe ourselves to be invincible. *Why wait for a locksmith when I can break the window?*

Chapter 5: Awakening

"Rock bottom" is one of the most familiar phrases to addicts. Typically, a rock bottom is the absolute lowest point of an addict's life—the moment when he or she realizes there is no other way but out. For one person, rock bottom might be landing in jail or facing bankruptcy; for another, it might be simply recognizing things cannot possibly get any worse for them. Many addicts die before reaching their personal rock bottom.

I emphasize the word personal when it comes to hitting rock bottom and sustaining recovery. Nobody else can identify or label our rock bottom; that is upon us. In my opinion, family and friends can help by allowing the addict to experience the consequences instead of shielding the hard truth. For example, if you are close to someone at work who's consistently late because of blacking out the night before, it's much better to allow your boss to punish this person than to cover for him or her.

If an addict has no consequences, they won't realize there is a problem. Not "protecting" an addict can be hard and counterintuitive, as it hurts to see a loved one suffer, but you will be doing them a big favor. One that could save their lives. Probably the easiest way to do this is to detach the disease and the manifestations of the disease from the person, and this is the quest I started when I had my awakening.

My awakening began immediately after the incident during my go-kart team outing—July 2014. The next day I went to work scared as hell to face everyone. *What could I possibly say; what were they going to think?* So, I acted as normal as I possibly could have, thanked everyone for their assistance and concern and mentioned that I got much better once I got home and rested. I knew most people would not buy it, but it was all I could conjure. I was lucky that I still had a job after that incident, so I wanted to keep as low of a profile as possible.

"I Am Different from All of Them"

I recall searching for AA meetings close to home and work and found a place a couple of miles away from my hotel which had a meeting every day at 5:30pm—it was a perfect opportunity. I called Laura scared from everything that had happened, confessed that I really needed help, and that I was going to attend an AA meeting. Throughout the previous months she had begun to comprehend that my drinking had gone far beyond having a blast and partying. As I began to open up about my challenges with alcohol, I could tell from our conversations that she had begun to realize it was a bigger issue than a simple choice to drink and have a good time. When I shared with her that I was going to an AA meeting, she was super supportive, and I could hear the relief in her voice as there was a glimpse of hope on stopping this madness.

I drove to the church where the meetings took place, and the parking lot was full. I felt like a little boy on the first day of school. I was scared, shy, and not quite sure how to act or what to do. I walked into the room, and there must have been 30 to 40 people from all walks of life. I immediately felt the positive vibe and welcoming atmosphere. I never had been in a place where everybody seemed to let down their guard without a word. Love filled the room.

At the beginning of AA meetings there is an opportunity for any newcomers or someone who is visiting from out of town to introduce themselves if they choose to do so. When I heard that, my heart was beating fast. I was anxious but I raised my hand to introduce myself: "Hi, I am Cesar, and I am an alcoholic." It felt weird saying it for the first time in my life. I was not sure if I believed in it or not, but I said it anyway.

The meeting I attended was an open discussion meeting. At an open discussion meeting, the chairperson begins the meeting with a topic of his or her choice and then opens up for discussion, so anyone is able to share their thoughts, experiences, or anything they choose to share related to the topic. I began looking around the room. *These people are actually not that weird – at least not all of them*, I thought. At that point in my life, I had not realized just how much all of us in the room had in common and felt more aligned with those who looked "normal" and professional like me than those who appeared to be poor and homeless. My bias and judgment were very much alive.

But as people began sharing their experiences, I immediately began noticing many similarities among our journeys and the thought processes, pain, anger, and resentment we felt—it was enlightening. It was refreshing to know that I was not alone and even though many of us had different backgrounds and life experiences, all of us shared a common ground. My judgment began to diminish slightly, as did my fear of opening up.

I realized during my first AA meeting that I was not going to achieve what I needed to unless I shared something. I had all this emotion and confusion inside my chest, and I needed to let it out. *If not here, then where? What a better and safer place to do so?* It was a room full of people who had been through or were going through similar situations to me. I built up my confidence and raised my hand to speak. I shared that I was tired of living a double life. I was tired of the pain I was feeling inside and causing my loved ones. I was a lucky person who had gotten away with it for a very long time. I'd had no real run-ins with the law and somehow no financial consequences. Amazingly enough I still had a beautiful family and a 3-year-old daughter who could still be proud of her dad. I knew that if I did not change my ways, sooner or later all of it would come to an end.

Wow—what a relief. It was like 10,000 pounds had been lifted off my shoulders. After the meeting, I got hugs and pats on the back from my fellow AA members. I felt and reciprocated a warmth that I haven't felt in a long time.

I continued to attend meetings as often as I could. I was more and more impressed about the non-judgmental approach strangers were having toward me and how much love they were giving me without asking or expecting anything in return. It was weird; I never thought a stranger could love you, but I was proven wrong; it was powerful.

But my ego still took hold. The more I began to learn about AA and the twelve steps through reading, meetings, and interactions with people, the more I began to compartmentalize the program into two sections: the parts that applied to Cesar and the parts that I could skip because I immediately "got" them or because they sounded a bit cultish to me.

I recall the thought of never having a drink again scaring me to death. *What do you mean I can never have a drink again? Would I never be able to get well and eventually manage my drinking as a normal person does?* (This is the obsession of every alcoholic.) These and many other thoughts came to mind, and they always led in one way or another to: *Most things in here do not apply to me because I am different from all of them—I may have my issues, but a lot of these people are really messed up.*

For the next 5 months I continued on this path. I was attending AA meetings and working on the steps with my sponsor—who is a fantastic person—on a selective basis just as I was choosing college classes. Of course, during this time, I kept saying whatever my sponsor and the AA people wanted to hear just as I had done with the therapist. During conversations with my fellow AA members, I would concur with whatever they said and repeat all the jargons and doctrine beliefs I heard in the rooms so they would not preach to me. I wanted to get out of AA what I thought I needed and keep my distance from the rest of it.

A Ticking Time Bomb

While I knew I had a problem and needed help I was still not 100% sold that I was a true alcoholic and that I would have to stay away from alcohol for the rest of my life. I was a walking, ticking time bomb and a relapse was just a matter of time.

December 19th, 2014. I was waiting on some news for a job I had recently interviewed for and that I really wanted. I was in a meeting when they called, so I let it go to voice mail. After the meeting was over, I listened to the message from the HR person saying that she wanted to speak to me when I was able to return her call.

That was it. I immediately jumped to the conclusion that I hadn't gotten the job. I was consumed by my emotions, negativity, and self-pity. After all, I thought, if I had the job, she would have said that in the message and congratulated me.

That was the trigger I needed to default to my old way of thinking and justification for drinking. I jumped into my car and headed to Publix, where I bought some wine and began to drink the first bottle in the parking lot.

Now that I was feeling the buzz, I felt prepared to call the HR lady back and hear the bad news. She answered the phone and said that she would like to offer me the job. I was in shock! She began reading the offer along with the benefits and asked me if I was interested in joining the company. *What? Did I just hear that right?* I was ecstatic! My sorrow and self-pity immediately turned into joy and happiness. I could not believe it! So now instead of drinking to forget and to numb my disappointment I was drinking for joy and celebration. I had my dream job. I finished the bottles of wine I had purchased, and then I went back to work and hit the hotel rooms to get some extra alcohol as the three bottles had not been enough. It was crazy.

At the end of the day, I got into my car and called Laura to tell her the news and let her know I was on my way home. She asked me if I was drunk. I broke down. I told her that I was very drunk; I was sorry that I was such a loser and wanted to die so I would not cause any more pain to her and Gabby. I was a failure. I don't remember much of our conversation, but I do remember her compassion. She was very reassuring. She said that it was okay, she realized that I was trying, and she would be there to help me. We would get through this together, but I needed to pull over and let her come and get me. I agreed to it and pulled over into a 7-Eleven a mile or two down the road from the hotel.

Laura was so lost and wasn't sure what to do. She asked me to stay put while she called my sponsor. That is the blessing of AA and its community. They will be there for you and your family no matter what. My sponsor talked my wife through the situation, explaining what to do, and kept her as calm as she could possibly be under the circumstances.

Our house was about 35 minutes from my work, so I had to sit in my car and wait. While Laura was on the phone with my sponsor, I was sitting in my car and then decided to go into 7-Eleven and buy a couple of the small bottles of wine to drink while I was waiting for her.

This was my rock bottom.

However, my rock bottom was also brightened by Laura's support and the peace I felt when she told me, *"Cesar, I know that you are trying to stop drinking and we will do this together."*

That was it—the sobriety switch flipped for me.

The next morning, we woke up early and she told me we were going to an AA meeting and that before the meeting we would meet with my sponsor and a couple of the other guys I knew. This was the best and most helpful thing all of them could have done for me—get me to face my decisions, my shame and fear while it was still very fresh. These guys had been around AA for several years and had seen it all. They had a heart-to-heart conversation with me and explained to me and Laura that nothing, nothing at all matters other than Cesar getting sober. It came before work, before family and anything else at this time. Without sobriety nothing else was possible.

Looking back, it's funny that one of my fuels to addiction (self-centeredness/selfishness) was one of the contributing factors to my sobriety path. Same quality, opposite application.

As we finished our coffee, we went to the AA meeting and Laura was by my side. It was a great and powerful meeting as I saw many of other AA members I knew from a different location, and some of them had come just to support me, which gave me hope. I was given another chance and I knew I had to embrace it. The love was contagious. From that day forward I unequivocally knew deep in my heart I could never have another drop of alcohol. I was 100% convinced and certain that there were no shortcuts and no other way. If I wanted to walk the walk and live a life of self-respect, health and rebuild the trust and connection with my family I would have to do this.

Biology and Environment: DNA and Triggers

Earlier I wrote about genetic variations and some of the testing I underwent in 2023. Having genetic errors in any of these genes can lead to a variety of health problems depending on the specific gene and the nature of the error. When multiple genes have genetic errors, the effects can be compounded, leading to a greater risk of developing certain health conditions. Armed with this information, I decided to dig a bit deeper and try to understand how having genetic errors in these and other genes may have had a direct impact in my predisposition to addiction.

I learned that there is evidence to suggest that genetic variations in the MAO-B, GAD1, HTR2A, and CoQ2 genes may be associated with an increased risk of addiction, although the mechanisms underlying these associations are not yet fully understood.

Genetic variations in the MAO-B gene, for example, have been linked to an increased risk of alcoholism and drug addiction. This may be because MAO-B is involved in the breakdown of dopamine, a neurotransmitter that plays a key role in the brain's reward system. Genetic variations in the MAO-B gene may alter dopamine levels, leading to changes in reward processing that increase the risk of addiction.

Similarly, genetic variations in the GAD1 gene have been associated with an increased risk of addiction, particularly in individuals with a family history of alcoholism – which is definitely my case. GAD1 is involved in the production of GABA, a neurotransmitter that is thought to play a role in the brain's reward system. Changes in GABA levels may alter the reward response to addictive substances, leading to an increased risk of addiction.

Genetic variations in the HTR2A gene have also been linked to an increased risk of addiction, particularly in individuals with a history of substance abuse. HTR2A is involved in the regulation of serotonin, a neurotransmitter that is thought to play a role in the brain's reward system. Changes in serotonin levels may alter the response to addictive substances, leading to an increased risk of addiction.

Moreover, genetic variations in the CoQ2 gene may also be linked to an increased risk of addiction, particularly in individuals with a family history of drug abuse. CoQ2 is involved in the production of CoQ10, a molecule that plays a role in cellular energy production. Changes in CoQ10 levels may affect the function of brain cells, altering the response to addictive substances.

It is important to note, that while genetic variations in these genes may increase the risk of addiction, they do not guarantee that an individual will develop an addiction. Many other factors, including environmental factors and individual differences in behavior and cognition, also play a role in the development of addiction.

Although I didn't find a single DNA cause for my addiction, I did discover that my genetic makeup played a significant role. It turns out that certain errors in my genetic code (SNPs) made me more susceptible to addiction if triggered by environmental factors. I always had a hunch that my DNA played a part, but now I have concrete evidence. The good news is that there are ways to mitigate these triggers and continue my path to better mental and physical health. It's reassuring to know that I have the power to suppress these genetic markers and take control of my well-being.

Powerful Lessons

- If an addict has no consequences, they won't realize there is a problem. Not "protecting" an addict can be hard and counterintuitive, as it hurts to see a loved one suffer, but you will be doing them a big favor.
- For addicts, the similarities among our journeys, thought processes, pain, and the anger and resentment we felt can be enlightening.
- There is evidence to suggest that genetic variations in the MAO-B, GAD1, HTR2A, and CoQ2 genes may be associated with an increased risk of addiction, although it is likely that other factors, including environmental factors and individual differences in behavior and cognition, may be required to develop addiction.

Part 2: The Four Pillars of Sobriety

"I am grateful that I found my wings before hitting the ground." – Mike Tyson

When I started writing this book in 2015, I was almost 10 months sober. This is what I wrote:

"Without a doubt it has been the best period of my life. I have begun to feel joy, happiness and a high from within. I found Cesar. The kind, warm, happy, and loving kid that has been inside all along.

There is still a long way to go in my recovery and I hope there are still many more great chapters to follow in my life and with my wonderful family. In a way, it almost feels like being born again. I have to re-learn how to feel emotions and channel it in a healthy way, I have to find new habits, a new routine and create a true circle of friends that I distanced myself from for many years while in isolation.

I have been given so many chances in my life. I certainly got more than my fair share. This is my time to show to myself and to many people suffering from addiction that recovery is possible. It is possible for everyone; no exceptions. Everyone has a different journey on how we got to this point, but all of us can have the same outcome of recovery. We just have to work for it.

I credit my recovery to many things; but I strongly believe there were some key aspects to it that have been crucial to me. I call it my four pillars of sobriety however I believe there are many applications for it in life regardless of someone's situation."

Today, as I revise this book for publication, I've discovered even more about the four pillars of sobriety, which I cover in the next four chapters.

Chapter 6: Acceptance

This sounds fairly simple and straightforward, which is just what I thought before my relapse.

Acceptance, while a simple word, is like a puzzle for an addict mind. I'd been lying to myself for so long that my fantasy world became reality to me. As I'd had no major consequences, I truly believed I had no issue with alcohol. My mind played tricks on me, I made excuses for every possible scenario, and I always had a justification for my drinking and behavior no matter how outrageous it was. No one can truly reach acceptance unless they have hit rock bottom. What is open for debate is what that means for each addict, as I wrote earlier in this book.

My rock bottom was relatively high, as I still had a job, a marriage, a clean record, and a dependable bank account. For others, rock bottom can mean several DUIs, loss of family and friends, becoming homeless, and prostitution among other possible outcomes. Some never hit their rock bottom before dying from their addiction.

I remember a story from one of my AA meetings that to me is a great example on how the mind of an addict works. This gentleman was telling the story of his first DUI. He got it on a fairly busy road in Ft. Lauderdale. Most people without an addiction problem would make sure to drastically reduce their drinking after a DUI and for sure never drive drunk again—but an addict thinks differently. His thought process on the next time he was about to drive drunk was: *I will go a different route. I will go through the back roads since they have a DUI trap on my usual route.* Who in their right mind would change the route they take to avoid a DUI instead of making the obvious choice of not driving drunk?

What I love about acceptance is that it will inadvertently lead to a crucial aspect needed for recovery: self-honesty. I am not saying that all recovering addicts are honest people and never lie. That is not the case, but unless you are honest with yourself about your addiction, you will never have a chance in recovery. You may not be ready to share or be completely honest with others about your drinking, but that may not matter as long as you are honest with yourself.

Self-honesty is a must for the recovery process. It requires addicts to acknowledge the extent of their addiction and its repercussions. Being honest with oneself involves dismantling the façades and facing the truth, even when it's uncomfortable or painful. It's a key step toward embracing change and seeking support.

In order to be ready to recover, I had to admit to myself that my life was in complete chaos, my way of life was not working anymore and that I was unable to manage it on my own. My best actions and thinking had led me to my personal rock bottom—clearly, I needed to open up to others and search for a different approach to my life. I fired myself from managing my own life.

Acceptance involves acknowledging the presence of addiction, understanding its impact on life, and then taking active steps toward change. But this process is often challenging because of denial, our fear of change, and the stigma associated with addiction.

Powerful Lessons

- Acceptance, while a simple word, is like a puzzle for an addict mind. We lie to ourselves for so long that our fantasy worlds become reality to us.
- Acceptance will inadvertently lead to a crucial aspect needed for recovery: self-honesty.
- Unless you are honest with yourself about your addiction, you will never have a chance in recovery. You may not be ready to share or be completely honest with others about your drinking, but that may not matter as long as you are honest with yourself.

Chapter 7: Gratitude

It's truly remarkable how one simple shift in mindset can change the course of your life. I've come to realize that placing gratitude at the center of everything we do can bring immense joy and fulfillment. I speak from experience—by acknowledging all the blessings in my life, from my health to my family to the opportunities that have come my way, I've discovered a sense of happiness that had eluded me for so long. It's a powerful lesson that I'll keep close to my heart forever. Little did I know that all these years, happiness was always inside of me and all I had to do is to let it be. Life got exponentially better. It is the best high of my life and for once a very healthy one.

For many years I was extremely ungrateful. I had consistently focused on what I did not have, and that I was not getting what I deserved. I became increasingly bitter and unhappy. Even though I was very fortunate and had so many blessings and good people and things around me, I chose to always default into a scarcity mindset, which was focused on negativity and became a self-fulfilling prophecy. I became a bottomless vortex of self-pity that was spiraling out of control. Gratitude saved me from this insanity and brought me to an inner peace that I desperately needed.

I am learning that being grateful will eventually bring you closer to God, or your higher power, whatever that might be for you. It is impossible to be truly grateful and not realize that there is a power greater than you.

You cannot be truly grateful while being self-centered; they are mutually exclusive qualities. I was very skeptical about acknowledging and believing in a higher power. I was an anti-religion crusader and incorrectly associated religion with spirituality.

As I continue to get clarity as time passes by with my sobriety, I am dropping my guard down and erasing my preconceived notions and anger towards spirituality. I am accepting that there is something greater than myself, and it is okay to open myself up and experience it. As I gained years of sobriety, it was no longer a sign of weakness but instead a sign of courage and humility to stop seeing myself as the center of the universe.

Everyone is just as important regardless of their struggles and what stage of the journey they find themselves. Everyone has a purpose in this life, and all purposes are equally important. Let me repeat it: *Everyone has a purpose in this life, and all purposes are equally important.*

In my experience, being grateful is not always easy and it takes practice. I've found many ways to cultivate gratitude in my daily life. One effective method is to write down the things we are thankful for each day. These can be as simple as a song we heard, a bird we saw, or something funny a child said to us. By practicing these daily affirmations, I have been able to better focus on positive aspects of my life. Being thankful encourages me to seek out more things to be grateful for. We can also express gratitude to others by writing thank-you notes or simply saying "thank you" more often.

While I am very grateful and have experienced a tremendous positive impact from it, I am just scratching the surface. This is a lifetime experience of awareness and humility that will lead me to nirvana.

Powerful Lessons

- Placing gratitude at the center of everything we do can bring immense joy and fulfillment.
- You cannot be truly grateful while being self-centered; they are mutually exclusive qualities.
- Everyone has a purpose, and all purposes are equally important.

Chapter 8: Community

I re-learned the meaning of community through AA. Throughout my years of addiction, I found myself more and more isolated. I changed as a person. I had been a young guy with lots of close and real relationships. I'd had a lot of close friends and was part of a large community. I gave all my energy to others and received it back 10 times more. As I began my journey to addiction, my personality and my brain changed. I metamorphosed into a dark and introverted person. I went from an extroverted class clown into a secluded, quiet person drifting away from everyone and everything. It was a lonely place but a place where Cesar was the king and the only voice to be heard. It felt great to always be right!

It is amazing how all the pillars of my recovery are interconnected. Without acceptance and gratitude, I could not have opened up to the concept of community and vice-versa. It was so refreshing and joyful to begin to feel other people's warmth and positive vibes. It is crazy how when you are isolated for such a long time, experiencing the simple things in life feels so good. I can only imagine how much better my life will continue to be as my community evolves.

Being part of a sober community in recovery has profound impacts. Acceptance, self-honesty, and gratitude make us humble, and a like-minded community reinforces that humility. We begin to see commonalities rather than differences. When we trust members of a community, we become vulnerable, and transparent, and we feel safe. While we are in addiction, and even at the beginning of our sobriety journey, we have the tendency to overthink, and to believe we can do anything, and control everything—these fallacies fall apart when we feel human connection in a community by letting our guard down.

Powerful Lessons

- Being part of a sober community in recovery has profound impacts.
- Acceptance, self-honesty, and gratitude make us humble, and a like-minded community reinforces that humility.
- When we trust members of a community, we become vulnerable, and transparent, and we feel safe.

Chapter 9: Healthy Habits

This pillar is hard. It feels like someone dropped you off in the middle of the desert and tells you to find home. *What do I do? How do I go about finding the right direction?* This is exactly how I felt once I quit drinking since all my activities revolved around alcohol. I was lost.

Thankfully, I have a great family that I love to spend time with and were thrilled to have me "back," so I was very lucky in that regard. I had an easy default to stay busy physically and mentally. Boredom is one of the most dangerous states of mind for a recovering addict. We can quickly begin to drift into the old thoughts, romanticize about that nice glass of cabernet over dinner and suddenly we are justifying how our old ways make sense. The busier we are, the less likely we are to have thoughts of drinking.

I quickly had to learn to avoid certain situations such as hanging out in bars or parties where drinking was an important part of it. Not because I would immediately default into drinking but what good could come out of it? Especially as a freshman in recovery. My first sponsor used to tell me, "You can't fail a test you don't take." Avoidance in this case was smarter and possibly more courageous than a possible false level of self-confidence. I have way too much to lose, and nothing will get in between myself and my sobriety—nothing.

A "weird" but fantastic healthy habit I had when I first became sober was chanting. It helped me get centered and focus on positive things. If I felt funny or if I was in a funk, chanting quickly brought me back to the gratitude lane. It gave me an opportunity to channel on a daily basis all the things that I was thankful for and allowed me to focus all my positive wishes and thoughts I had for myself, my family and the world. It worked.

As my sobriety journey evolved, so did my healthy habits. While I enjoyed the chanting for a while, I explored other habits from exercises, reading, and several others. As of now, I believe I have found a couple of them I will stick with for a little while. It is a daily morning affirmation, a 12-minute guided daily affirmation that has truly been transformative to me. I have done it for more than a year and a half as I write this book at the end of 2023, and I have experience tangible growth and progress in my life because of it. From a physical aspect over the last two years, I have been fairly consistent on staying active, and a recent habit I have been developing is the proacting of Jiu-Jitsu. I am a novice, and don't know much but just by practicing and rolling with my classmates it is like therapy to me. It is a time that all my worries, stress and thoughts are dissipated. It is a great exercise for my mind and body (despite some bruising and minor injuries from time to time ☺)

Writing has been another healthy habit to keep me in the moment. This is a very unexpected one as I was never great in writing or enjoy writing as you can probably conclude from my poor performance as a student early in my life. However, once I began writing not because I was asked to and began to write simple things such as my thoughts, ideas, and write gratitude it was a wonderful discovery. It feels great to be writing this book and as the years progressed, I began writing blogs as well—I would never have thought in a million years that I would be capable of this or would want to do it. A great reminder to never say never or limit yourself. I am not sure how people will perceive my book and how much it will make sense to readers, but without a doubt it has been a therapeutic experience for me. Through this process I have been able to reflect, learn and fuel my recovery. It has been a fantastic experience!

With the hope of reaching out to anyone affected by addiction, I have felt a deep desire to share a part of my personal journey. Whether it is someone struggling with addiction themselves, a concerned loved one or simply a curious teenager, I wanted to shed light on this difficult topic. If my story can offer even a glimmer of hope or understanding to someone, then it will all have been worthwhile. Let's all work towards supporting each other in overcoming addiction, one day at a time.

Powerful Lessons
- Boredom is one of the most dangerous states of mind for a recovering addict.
- "You can't fail a test you don't take." Avoiding certain situations is one of the simplest healthy habits an addict early in recovery can adopt.

- Let's all work towards supporting each other in overcoming addiction, one day at a time.

Part 3: The Powers of Addiction

"Out of suffering have emerged the strongest souls; the most massive characters are seared with scars." — Kahlil Gibran

What a journey it has been these past nine years since I first began writing this book. Thankfully, as I write this my life has become continuously better in many ways, including a much closer relationship with my wife Laura, and daughter Gabby (now 13) which was the catalyst for my desire to begin and maintain my sobriety.

Being sober for this long has been an incredible milestone that brings a sense of pride, accomplishment, and a renewed appreciation for life. This journey of self-discovery and personal growth has been transformative and has led to improvements in every aspect of my life, from personal relationships to health, happiness, and professional success.

As you know by now, my decision and path to become sober was not an easy one. It came after a lot of turns, infliction of pain for my loved ones and self-harm, but it was a necessary journey that has allowed me to find my inner self again. Alcohol had become a crutch that I relied on to numb my emotions, avoid dealing with difficult situations, and to escape from reality.

Upon reflection, the first few months of sobriety were challenging as I had to relearn how to cope with life's stressors without relying on alcohol. But as time went on, I noticed the positive changes in my life, which has given me the desire to stay focused on what matters most and avoid giving in to temptations. As time passed by, I started to feel more present, more clear-headed, and more in control of my emotions. I found that I had more energy and motivation to tackle my daily tasks and pursue my goals.

While I am proud of my achievement thus far, a lot of questions remain from when I first began writing this book. While I know that my biology, environment, development, and choices I made contributed to becoming an addict I still wonder how much each part has played. I guess I won't be able to get a report card showing all the details and percentages of each contributing factor along with a timeline ☺.

Was I destined to become an addict, or were the choices I made ultimately the reason for it? After nine years I am still revisiting these questions in search of an answer. The good news is that I have enough understanding now to know that it was not only a bad intention or desire within me, but several things that together created the perfect environment to becoming an addict.

My reasons to search for answers were twofold: first, to satisfy my own curiosity; and second, to help my daughter Gabby gain insight into the illness that plagued her father. Armed with knowledge, she could make informed decisions that might prevent her from straying down the same treacherous path I once walked. I want to break the cycle! As a parent, nothing is more heartbreaking than seeing your child in pain. That's why I'm on a mission to do everything in my power to help my daughter. I know that I caused my family a lot of pain in the past, but now I'm determined to turn that pain into something positive. I want to use my experiences to learn, grow and hopefully make things right—even though I know I can never fully make up for my mistakes.

The second reason for this search is to empower not only myself but also other addicts with the knowledge that can turn our biggest failures, our deepest sorrows, and our most intense pain into our greatest triumphs, our highest joys, and our most liberating relief. Because the same forces that contribute to our addiction are the same ones that turn us into better people, parents, friends, workers, and contributors to society. These are the powers of addiction.

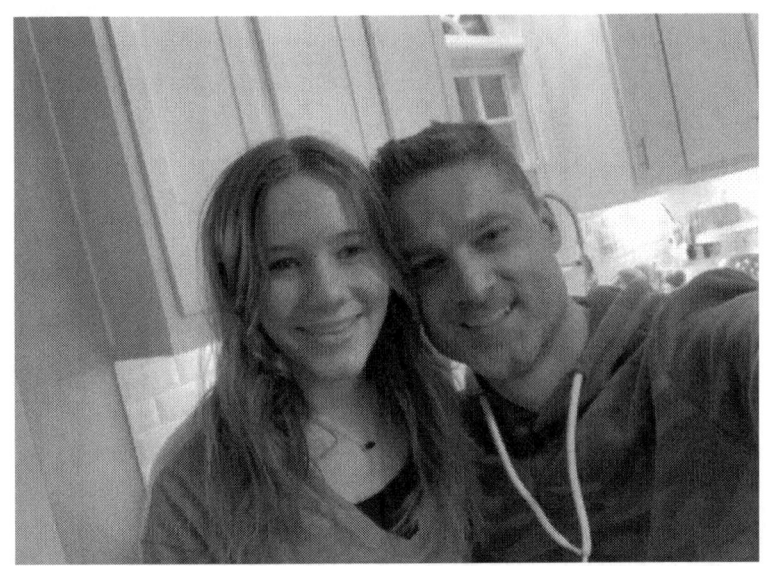

Me and Gabby on the morning of my 8th year of sobriety. A proud moment for us as a family!

Chapter 10: Family Influences

The trauma of losing my mom was a tremendous influence. Burying my grief after her death, I've discovered, contributed to my struggles with addiction. As long as I did not have to feel and deal with the pain of losing my mom, life was better. Once I mastered suppressing the feeling of loss, doing the same with future struggles became a habit and easier as time went by. My mastering of this skill was facilitated by not having an outlet to share my emotions, at home or anywhere else, and the easiest way to avoid my feelings was to numb them with alcohol.

Growing up with a father who battled addiction was another challenging environment factor that I attribute to my journey to addiction. We now know that I have inherited genetic variations linked to impulse control and the brain's reward system that increase my likelihood of addiction. Even though I didn't experience any major traumatic events because of my father's addiction, the little traumas throughout the years due to the constant sense of fear and lack of safety posed a frequent daily challenge.

Alcohol impacts more than addicts. As I've written throughout this book, it has a tremendous impact on almost everything an addict touches. And even for non-addicts, society's acceptance and celebration of alcohol can be deadly. It is surreal to learn the impact and ramifications that alcohol has in many people's lives. One does not necessarily have to be alcoholic or a heavy drinker to suffer serious consequences from this drug.

Ronald

Laura and I recently learned that her father, Ronald (Ron), has liver cancer.

My father in-law is not an alcoholic, but it seems that the accumulation of 40-plus years of drinking on a somewhat frequent basis has caught up with him. We trust our doctors to catch problems when we have regular check-ups, but alcohol's effects can be missed by a system built to trust or ignore people when they dismiss their alcohol consumption as a glass or two of wine a week.

Ron had reported a few symptoms such as a bloated stomach and loss of weight, but after his doctor ran tests, Ronald was simply given the advice to watch his diet.

Misleading test results (such as no abnormality in liver enzymes if your liver has cirrhosis) can add to the misconception and naiveness that many people have about drinking and the harm it causes to our body. This is the danger when as society we normalize the use of a drug that is expected to be self-controlled.

How could this have happened? After all, Ronald was going every six months to the doctor and had all the traditional physical exams and blood work done, in addition to getting a specific test that shows abnormalities and the possibility of cancer in his body. All these tests up to most recently—less than 6 months ago, as I write—showed no abnormality or anything unusual about his liver or cancer. As a matter of fact, his liver enzymes show to be normal even right now as he lays in the hospital.

When the doctor at the hospital came to tell Ronald about the liver cancer, he told him that when you have cirrhosis, your liver does not produce enzymes therefore results can come back normal. This was a shock to all of us. Why do we rely on tests if they can be so misleading?

As a matter of fact, when I was drinking a lot of my measurement of how bad my drinking was, was based on my liver test results. When it used to come within normal ranges—which was the vast majority—I justified to myself that my drinking couldn't be that bad. With this type of self-diagnosis on the impact of drinking we are playing with fire. How could I be abusing alcohol if my body was handling it?

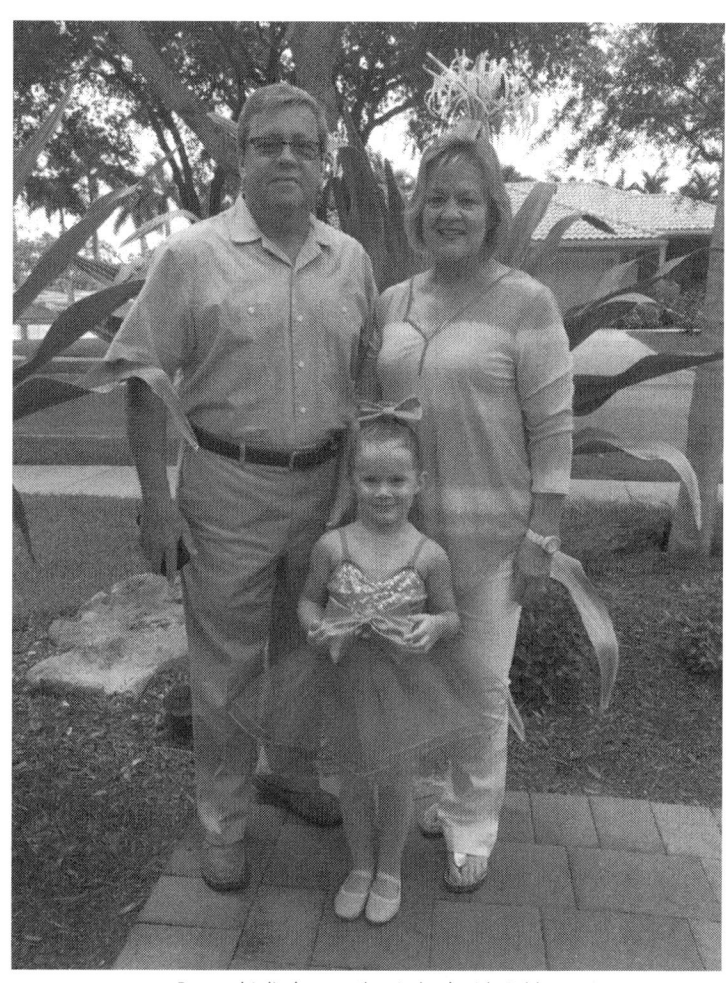

Ron and Julie (my mother in-law) with Gabby

My Dad

Unfortunately, my dad never stopped drinking or decided to get help for his addiction. He kept drinking as usual, perhaps a little less, but nevertheless, kept drinking every day and as much as he could. A turning point on his drinking and overall health happened when my dad retired many years ago. When he was let go of his job, which forced his retirement, his self-esteem and self-worth took a big hit. He stayed down, never took interest in acquiring hobbies, spending time with friends, or even taking a little walk around the neighborhood. He was always at home watching TV and drinking. Even reading newspapers, which was one of his favorite things to do when I was growing up, was no longer a hobby.

By living this sedentary life, his health deteriorated. For the most part, his physical health remained OK, but his brain started to suffer. Many years ago, we noticed that he was losing memory, and even a little bit of self-care and hygiene which had never been an issue for him. We came to find out that he had Alzheimer's, a disease that like addiction affects not only the patient but also their loved ones. It can be a devastating experience. The initial signs of memory loss and forgetfulness may seem minor, but as the disease progresses, the impact becomes more evident. It's heartbreaking to watch someone you care about struggle with the loss of their memory at an alarming rate. It is an experience I wouldn't wish on anyone. Watching my dad live with Alzheimer's is confusing and painful. He can't remember that he has two sons, was once married to my mom or that his loving wife of nearly three decades is the woman caring for him. In his mind, she's his sister, Claudia.

This experience has been extremely difficult, especially in the beginning—to realize that my dad, the dad I knew, was no longer there. However, I came to accept the progression of the disease. It's a challenging reality to face, but my family and I are determined to make the most of every moment we have left with him. When it comes to connecting with my dad, I've learned to be flexible and open-minded. I've noticed that sometimes he can get a little frazzled or lost, so I do my best to keep things calm and relaxed. It's all about making sure he feels comfortable and secure, even if that means going with the flow and embracing the unexpected. I also focus on talking about things that bring him joy. Even though we don't have the traditional father-son talks, we still have great conversations and to me, that is very special. My ultimate mission is to ensure that his remaining time on this planet is overflowing with joy and contentment. I am wholeheartedly committed to contributing to this cause in any way that I can.

A few years ago, reaching the age of 40 brought about a pivotal moment in my relationship with my dad. For years, I held onto anger and resentment towards him, focusing on our differences and the things he did that I disagreed with. It wasn't until later in life, and going through my own recovery journey and personal growth that I realized the importance of acceptance and forgiveness. Despite our flaws and disagreements, my dad is a wonderful person at heart, with a protective mindset and a deep love for his family. When I turned 40, I finally mustered the courage to tell him that I loved him for the first time. It wasn't easy, but it was necessary to let go of all the negative emotions that were only hurting me and keeping us apart. Looking back on it now, I am grateful that I took that step, as it allowed us to mend our relationship.

Have you ever noticed that seeing someone display the traits you despise about yourself can bring out a strong reaction in you? In my case, watching my dad reminded me of a part of myself that I tried to hide for many years. It was difficult to acknowledge and accept my own flaws and imperfections. By letting down my guard and showing my affection, I was able to be more accepting of him.

However, despite our progress, we were never able to achieve a deep, open connection. It was hard for him to fully grasp the commitment I had to sobriety, as he couldn't fathom life without alcohol. I am at peace knowing that both of us did the best we could — and that's what life is all about.

Powerful Lessons

- It is surreal to learn the impact and ramifications that alcohol has in many people's lives. One does not necessarily have to be alcoholic or a heavy

drinker to suffer serious consequences from this drug.
- Misleading test results can add to the misconception and naiveness that many people have about drinking and the harm it causes to our body. This is the danger when as society we normalize the use of a drug that is expected to be self-controlled.
- Have you ever noticed that seeing someone display the traits you despise about yourself can bring out a strong reaction in you? In my case, watching my dad reminded me of a part of myself that I tried to hide for many years.

Chapter 11: Choices

Choices. This is a puzzling one for me. While I know that may choices have played a significant part in me becoming an addict, I don't exactly know what the precise factor of its influence was, as well as the speed in which it contributed that I became one. However, I know how much choice followed by action is 100% the reason why and how I stay sober.

Addicts don't choose to be addicts. I never met an addict who strived to become one and chances are you haven't either. However, we know that the choices we make based on our DNA and environment will have a significant impact on someone's journey to addiction.

In today's society, there's a tendency to oversimplify matters related to choice. It's a common belief that a person with a good heart won't intentionally hurt others, and this logic is often mistakenly applied to addiction as well. However, this isn't accurate. While making good choices plays a role in preventing problems, it's not the only factor. Our ego and decision-making can become clouded, leading even those with the best intentions to consciously cause harm. Similarly, choosing to drink responsibly doesn't guarantee immunity from addiction. The reality is that numerous factors can influence such situations, making them far more complex than a mere matter of choice.

This isn't about making excuses or letting anyone off the hook. Choice plays a crucial role in addiction and in the recovery process; everyone has the option to seek help and strive for sobriety. Commitment and perseverance are essential. My own path to sobriety hasn't been straightforward, which is a common experience for many addicts. Therefore, an important aspect of making a choice is the resilience to get up when you fall, to persist and not surrender when faced with setbacks. By having a true north and staying committed to it no matter what, I found not only my sobriety but also my superpowers from all my hardships throughout my life. The below excerpt is from one of my earliest blog posts, written in April 2023. I selected it for inclusion in this section of the book because I found it very relevant and fitting.

"Life can be a wild ride, full of unexpected twists, turns, and bumps in the road. Whether it's financial woes, heartbreak, health setbacks, or any other type of challenge, we've all been there in some shape or form. While these tough times can be gut-wrenching and agonizingly difficult, they can also teach us valuable lessons about ourselves and the world around us. We emerge from these struggles stronger, wiser, and more equipped to help others facing similar hardships.

"Have you ever considered what your struggles have given you? I was inspired by a recent podcast featuring Jay Shetty and Ed Mylett where they explored the power of cultivating positive values. Their insights left a lasting impression on me, particularly the idea that our past hardships can actually be our greatest strength. From bankruptcy to addiction battles and everything in between, the challenges we face have the potential to shape us into a powerful force for good in the world. Reflecting on my own journey, I realized that my own struggles have gifted me with an unexpected superpower. So, let me ask you this—what unwanted superpowers have your struggles given you?

"Let's face it, no one actively seeks out hardships or tough times. But there's no denying that those struggles can lead to incredible growth and personal development. I remember when I was just 12 years old, losing my mom unexpectedly. It was a dark and difficult time for me and my family. However, that hardship forced me to learn and understand things at a young age that I otherwise wouldn't have. In fact, I consider them my superpowers.

"The painful loss of a loved one can profoundly affect our outlook on life. It has the ability to shift our priorities and bring into focus the fragility of our existence. Through personal experience, I've come to realize that such devastation can awaken a newfound appreciation for the present moment and the people we share it with. Surviving adversity can inspire us to live with more purpose and meaning, fueled by the understanding that life is precious and fleeting.

"Choosing to overcome hardships can actually help us become more resilient, and in turn, better able to support others who are dealing with difficult situations. By facing tough circumstances head-on, we develop coping mechanisms and skills that prepare us to come out stronger and more resourceful. And as we grow in our own resilience, we gain valuable experience that can help us guide and support those around us who might be going through similar struggles. Ultimately, our ability to overcome adversity can inspire and uplift others, and we can use our own trials and tribulations to offer hope and guidance to those in need.

"The saying goes that 'What doesn't kill you makes you stronger,' and it seems that this rings true when it comes to empathy and compassion. Those who have been through tough times understand the struggles of others going through similar situations and are often motivated to reach out and help them. By building connections with those who have shared similar experiences, we can enhance our own wellbeing—and create a more compassionate world in the process.

"After enduring challenging circumstances, we can come out on the other side with a newfound appreciation for life. Rather than solely focusing on our own problems, we gain a broader perspective that allows us to see the world in a more positive light. This altered view can be a powerful tool when supporting others who are also facing adversity. Suddenly, we can see the world in a more positive light and appreciate all that's good around us. And this perspective goes beyond just helping ourselves—it equips us with the tools to uplift others and offer them hope in their own struggles.

"When we face tough circumstances in life, it can feel like an insurmountable challenge. However, it's worth noting that these struggles can actually become opportunities for us to blossom and evolve. We can make the choice to turn pain into purpose. Tough experiences can motivate us to become more adaptable, absorb important teachings, cultivate a stronger sense of compassion, and recognize our own courage that lies within."

If you're interested in exploring and listening to the mentioned podcast episode, 'Ed Mylett ON: How to Break Down Your Goals Into Achievable Steps & Simple Ways to Create Positive Daily Habits, On Purpose with Jay Shetty,' you can find it on several platforms, including Apple Podcasts, Podtail, and Global Player, among others.

Powerful Lessons

- Addicts don't choose to be addicts. I never met an addict who strived to become one and chances are you haven't either.
- After enduring challenging circumstances, we can come out on the other side with a newfound appreciation for life.
- We can make the choice to turn pain into purpose.
- What superpowers have your struggles given you?

Chapter 12: Inner Nirvana

Gratitude, resilience, empathy, and hope! This is what my sobriety journey has taught me.

Reflecting on these values of gratitude, resilience, empathy, and hope that my journey to sobriety has instilled in me, I find myself contemplating the broader societal challenges related to alcohol. While I have gained much personally, I recognize that the battle against alcohol abuse extends beyond individual experiences. I'm uncertain about any significant changes in our healthcare system or in legislation concerning alcohol and its impact on society.

Deep down, I must admit, I'm not very optimistic about meaningful progress in these areas to effectively control alcohol, or in efforts to educate about, prevent, or treat abuse. However, I'm quite hopeful about the potential of individual and community efforts to improve and support each other. There's a growing desire to enhance personal well-being and care, which is certainly a cause for celebration. Looking at the newer generations, I see a much deeper awareness that instills in me hope for sustainable progress.

Engaging in open conversations about mental health, substance abuse, and life struggles can lay the foundation for a supportive and compassionate community. It takes courage to be vulnerable, but the reward is a safe space where individuals feel empowered to seek help and improve their well-being. By becoming more vulnerable I have greatly benefited in my recovery journey, and it also has paved the way for me to help others through collective growth and progress towards leading the best life possible. It has been heartwarming to make a lot of new connections, reconnect with old acquaintances and discover how deeply this topic impact almost everyone in this word; directly or indirectly.

When I shared my first book draft with some close friends and acquaintances, the response was resoundingly uplifting. In a world where addiction is often shrouded in shame and secrecy, they were grateful for my unfiltered account of my own trials and tribulations. Many praised my courage and bravery for revealing such personal insights and found it enlightening to witness someone lay bare their struggles so candidly. But the most rewarding feedback of all came from those who confided that my book had inspired them to pursue sobriety themselves. Though I could never take credit for their life-changing decisions, it's incredibly gratifying to know that my tale could serve as a positive impetus for others. I am cheering them on in their journey towards recovery with strength and resilience! This experience also reaffirms my belief in the power of sharing our stories. You never know how a simple act of sharing can impact someone's life. Your story, too, has the potential to inspire change!

After nine years, I am finally ready to transform this project into a book. As I began to write it, it started as a book but deep down I am not so sure I had the intent of ever publishing it. The fear of failure and self-doubt had me convinced that perhaps it would not be good enough, and maybe it will fail. Even now, those fears still linger. But I've learned to embrace them and understand that these are self-inflicted. I know that making this dream into reality will be challenging, but the possibilities are limitless especially if it helps save lives.

Upon receiving feedback from my book draft, I was comforted to realize that my work's worth isn't defined by book sales or media attention. Rather, it's about positively impacting people's lives, and the possibility of having them pay it forward by impacting others. This can be an everlasting chain that will outlive me.

The fundamental four pillars of acceptance, gratitude, community, and healthy habits still hold true even as I continue to grow and evolve. These pillars continue to provide me with a grounding effect that helps me stay focused on what matters most in life while keeping my sobriety at the forefront of it.

One of my passions in life became helping others. I have been blessed with a beautiful life and I see it as my duty to pay it forward. I am focused on bringing hope, kindness, and positive energy to this world and helping others with addiction—either directly or indirectly. Most recently I am accomplishing it through my LinkedIn posts, blogs, community engagement and being an advocate in the Diversity, Equity, and Inclusion (DE&I) space.

My journey towards sobriety began with two crucial ingredients: self-awareness and self-honesty. Once I found the courage to look inward, I was able to embrace forgiveness and understanding towards myself and others, unlocking my heart and soul to a world of possibility. I never dreamed of how great my life is today and all the wonderful things that happened over the last nine years. Through the power of self-worth and the unwavering support of my loved ones, I was able to find and hold onto an inner sense of Nirvana.

I hope you find yours too!

Let's Connect

LinkedIn   Blog

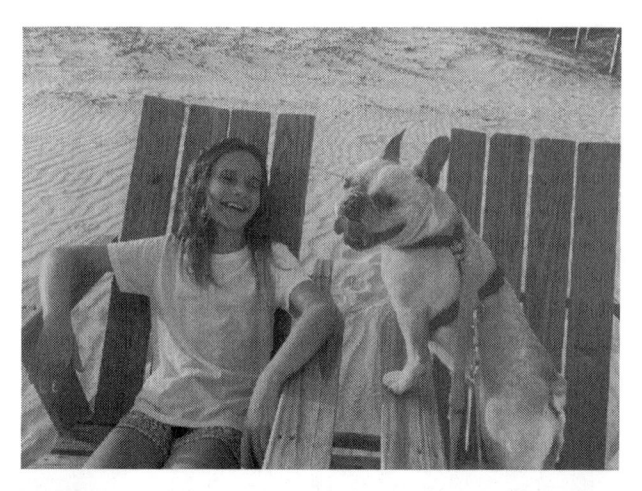

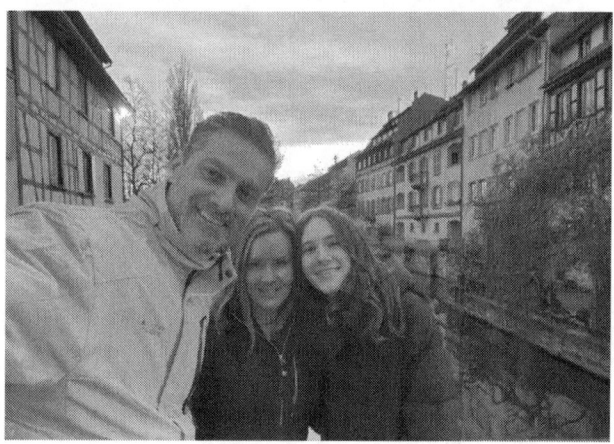

Gabby and Mila at the beach and a recent family vacation where the annoying part for the family was how I pretended to speak French vs. being hammered 😊

140

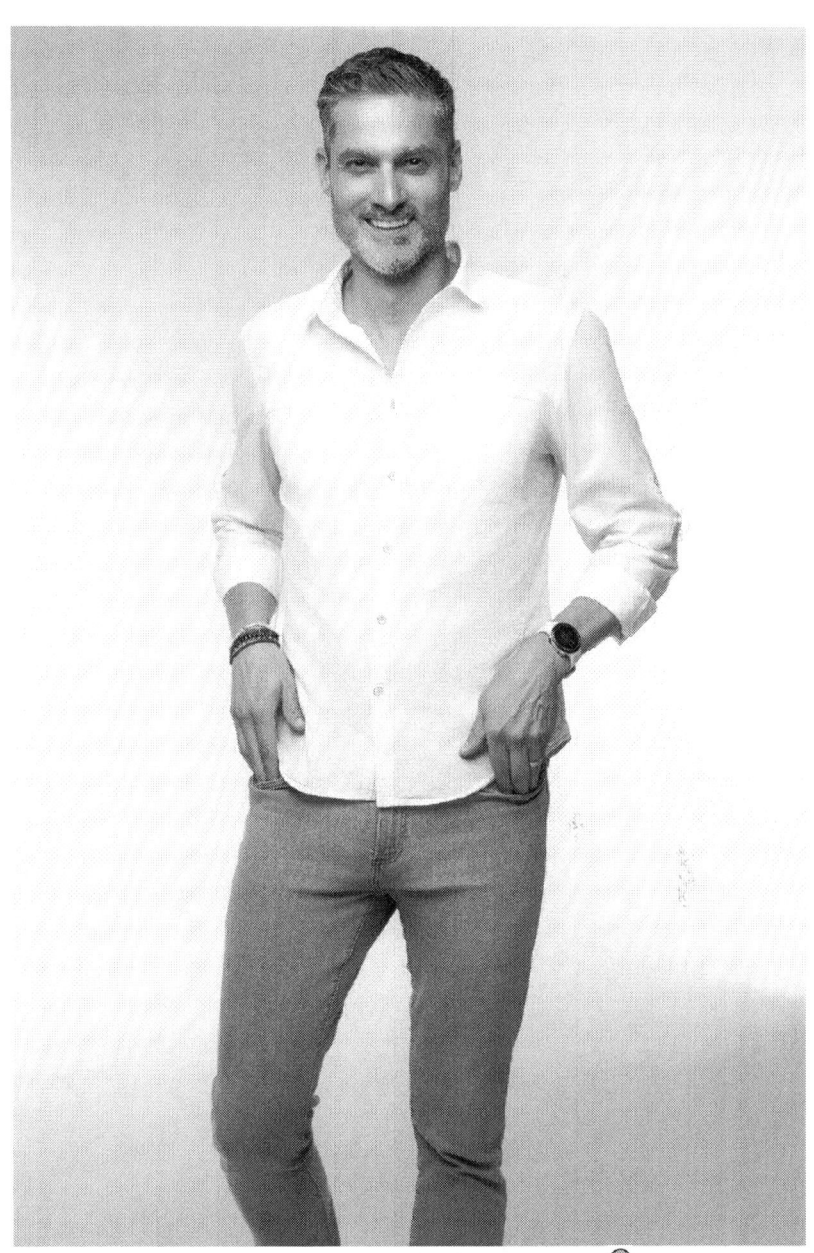

9 years sober! Photoshoot to figure out my book cover 😊

Made in the USA
Middletown, DE
25 April 2024